Quality Assurance Implementation in Research Labs

Akshay Anand
Editor

Quality Assurance Implementation in Research Labs

Springer

Editor
Akshay Anand
Department of Neurology
Neuroscience Research Lab
Post Graduate Institute of Medical Education and Research
Chandigarh
India

CCRYN Collaborative Centre for Mind Body Interventions by Yoga
Post Graduate Institute of Medical Education and Research
Chandigarh
India

ISBN 978-981-16-3073-6 ISBN 978-981-16-3074-3 (eBook)
https://doi.org/10.1007/978-981-16-3074-3

This Springer imprint is published by the registered company Springer Nature Singapore Pte Ltd.
The registered company address is: 152 Beach Road, #21-01/04 Gateway East, Singapore 189721, Singapore

Foreword

This book will be a guide for students and professionals alike in quality assurance practices related to clinical research labs. The historical research and fundamental principles make it a good tool in clinical research environments. The country has a great need for such a compilation in order to increase the application of domestic capabilities and technology.

Ratan N. Tata
TATA TRUSTS

Contents

1 **Historical Overview of Quality Assurance in Biological Research** 1
Radhika Khosla and Vinod Srivastava

2 **Conceptual Framework of Research Data Auditability** 15
Rahul Tyagi and Venkatesh Thuppil

3 **Management of Skilled Human Resources by Youth-Oriented Good Laboratory Practices (YOG)** 31
Sheetal J Gupta and Ajay Kumar Sehgal

4 **Operationalization of Research SOPs for PhD Scholars** 45
Priya Mehra, Gillipsie Minhas, and Winston Costa Pereira

5 **Creating Data Recording Sheets (DRS) in Quality Management System** 63
Manjari Rain, Madhava Sai Sivapuram, Deepali Mathur, and K. Sadasivan Pillai

6 **The Value of Master Schedules in Benchmarking Research Productivity** 79
Pranay Mahajan, Shweta Modgil, and Vipin Koushal

7 **Logsheets and the Academic Progress of Ph.D. Students** 95
Kalyan Maity and K. Sadasivan Pillai

8 **Instigation and Adherence to the Quality Assurance Program to Avoid Academic Conflicts** 113
Priya Battu, Bhavya Mody, Sumit Rana, and Kaushal Sharma

9 **Data Fraud and Essence of Data Verifiability** 137
Parul Bali, L. V. Simhachalam Kutikuppala, Pramod Avti, and Bikash Medhi

10 **The Role of Document Control and Archiving Records in Laboratory Management** 161
Navneet Kaur, Prashant Verma, Bhavya Mody, Neeru Malik, Gurmeet Singh, and Chirayu Padhiar

11 Academic Social Responsibility and Quality Assurance in the Developing World: A Framework for Implementation 181
Avijit Banik and Avik Mitra

12 Good Laboratory Practices: Lab Orientations, Meetings, and Value of Communication 193
Pooja Nadholta, Saras Jyoti, Sriloy Mohanty, Amit Singh, Jaideep Arya, and Neel Kamal Sharma

13 Role of Data Digitization on Data Integrity 221
Kanupriya Sharma, Vyas M. Shingatgeri, and Surinder Pal

About the Editor

Akshay Anand works as a Professor at Neuroscience Research Lab, Department of Neurology, and Prof in Charge, CCRYN Collaborative Center for Mind Body Interventions by Yoga, PGIMER, Chandigarh. He is an Adjunct Professor, Centre for Phenomenology and Cognitive Sciences, Department of Philosophy, Punjab University, Chandigarh and an Editor in Chief of Annals of Neurosciences and Integrative Medicine Case Reports (JIMCR) and a former EIC of Integrative Medicine International. He has 203 publications in international peer-reviewed journals (including 30 Policy research commentaries) besides filing four patent applications. He has mentored 14 PhD students and completed 20 research grants and remains profusely funded by various national funding agencies, advising various editorial, policy, and scientific enterprises across 30 countries. His research interests range from understanding of neuronal cell survival mechanisms using in vitro, in vivo, genetic, and alternative approaches (mindfulness techniques) to discovering biomarkers of neurodegenerative disorders for clinical applications. His research lab is the only research lab in India to voluntarily operationalize a voluntary Quality Assurance regimen duly recognized by the Quality Council of India. He serves as a Visiting Professor of the Kyoto University of Medicine and S-VYASA, Bengaluru and earlier also served with Lesya Ukrainian Eastern European National University, Lutsk and Sri Sri Institute of Advanced Research, Bengaluru as its Visiting Professor/Visiting Scientist. Dr. Anand was nominated for India's prestigious Padma Award, 2020 besides being honored by UT Police for exemplary work in advancement of Yoga research. He has been awarded for ICMR Amrut Mody Unichem Prize-2012, Annual PGI Faculty Award-2013, 2014, Sardar Vallabhbhai Patel Foundation 9th International Prestigious Sardar Patel Award, 2014, Scopus Young Scientist Award Runner up, National Academy of Sciences India, New Delhi, 2012, ICMR Shakuntala Amir Chand Award (2010), Young Scientist Award from DAE (2005), Retina Research Foundation/Joseph M. and Eula C. Lawrence Award (2003). He is also an Advisory Board Member, Harvard University, Boston, USA and an advisor of Research Activities in Sivananda Yoga Vedanta Academy, Bhubaneswar. He is also a Member of Academic and Administrative Committee, Center of Phenomenology and Cognitive Sciences-2021. His academic social activities like PM's Clean India program and "yoga scholars PGIMER" have cultivated an increased sense of preventive healthcare among his students, colleagues, and science practitioners.

Historical Overview of Quality Assurance in Biological Research

1

Radhika Khosla and Vinod Srivastava

1.1 Introduction

Quality Assurance, as suggested by its name, is a criterion to measure and to assure the quality in the production of goods and services. The users or customers demand good quality in goods and services. The need and demand for quality have always been there since human civilization originated. The most ancient concept of quality has been found during the Middle Ages when guilds [1] were formed to inspect the quality of products produced by blacksmiths, artisans, craftsmen [2], and merchants [1–9]. Guilds were a group of individuals of a particular trade who were experts in that trade. Experts analyzed the quality of products produced by other members or nonmembers of the guilds. Medical men were also known as medical crafts, although they did not like to be considered tradesmen. Humphreys has mentioned the concept of Guild medicine in the editorial [10, 11]. It used to be a matter of pride to be a member of guilds. Guild members were required to be highly skilled in their work to remain as a member of guilds. They had to create a profession-specific masterpiece to sustain affiliation or membership of the guilds. In the medieval times, there were several prime examples of steps taken to ensure the quality of products and their efficiency, such as William Wrotham's appointment to assess ships' quality during the emperorship of King John of England [12], and Secretary to the British Admiralty, Samuel Pepys' attempt to bring the quality in the

R. Khosla
Neuroscience Research Lab, Department of Neurology, Post Graduate Institute of Medical Education and Research, Chandigarh, Chandigarh, India

V. Srivastava (✉)
College of Health and Behavioral Sciences, Fort Hays State University, Hays, KS, USA
e-mail: vksrivastava@fhsu.edu

A. Anand (ed.), *Quality Assurance Implementation in Research Labs*,
https://doi.org/10.1007/978-981-16-3074-3_1

production of ships. Guilds were active and retained their place in history until the nineteenth century [3, 4, 12, 13]. However, these guilds started hindering free trade in the later stages that brought them toward their end.

In the early nineteenth century, the industrial revolution took place, and the mode of production changed. The rapid change in society from agrarian to industrial marked the shift in human resources, management styles, and industrial appropriations. Factories diluted the concept of guilds and gave prominence to foremen appointed in the factories to assess the quality of products manufactured in factories [3, 5]. The Industrial Revolution period marked the era of mass production, giving rise to the building of knowledge and expertise in quality assurance and quality control over the years [5]. This period can be divided into various eras [3].

1.2 Taylorian Era

Frederick Winslow Taylor is known as the father of scientific management [14–16] and the first consulting engineer in management [5, 17]. He was the pioneer of a new profession and brought scientific procedures into manufacturing to streamline productivity and efficiency. It was also called Taylorism in the name of its founder, Frederick Winslow Taylor, and was the hallmark of the progressive era [18]. The progressive era rejecting social Darwinism believed efficiency and productivity could help address social problems as well [18]. Taylor's goal was to enhance productivity in factories to a considerable level and used engineering plans and theories in management. Although there were strong protests from labor unions against efficiency and productivity in factories, the marriage of craftsmanship and quality was inevitable. However, the focus revolved primarily around the management of human resources than the processes.

The World War I factories were burdened with the demand to produce large quantities of goods. Craftsmen followed the engineers' plan and product requirements to meet the specifications of goods, but meeting the high demand of goods with the specific quality or relatively good quality started drawing management attention to process management [5]. As a result, the process of manufacturing started being invigilated [19]. However, as operation magnified and production increased, it became less feasible to ensure the quality of products. As a result, factories compromised quality for high production, and the rift between quality and quantity in management continued.

1.3 The Era of Quality Control (the 1920s)

In the mid-1920s, Walter Shewhart, a physicist and a statistician, began his work on improving the quality of industrial production. He was working at Bell Laboratories, and in around the 1930s, Shewhart gave the concept of

Plan-Do-Study-Act (PDSA) [20], which later came to be known as Plan-Do-Check-Act (PDCA) in Deming's era [16] of quality management, or Shewhart cycles [20]. This was the first time cycles were introduced in the quality control process, emphasizing process management, and thereafter the concept of lean production followed.

Shewhart introduced statistical procedures into quality checks to maintain the quality of products [19]. This concept was known as *Statistical Quality Control* [21], and Shewhart is known as the Father of Statistical Quality Control or Father of Modern Quality Control [4, 16]. Growth in industrialization and demand for mass production rendered quality control a tedious and cumbersome task, as checking the quality of every product being produced in a factory or organization was not feasible. Tools of statistical quality control provided inspectors and quality control managers with some statistical measures to assess the quality of mass production. Product sampling and control charts were used to compare and assess the quality of the products [22]. Standard Statistical tools provided production houses with the confidence of quality in their products. During the World War II, the US Army did not want to compromise quality with mass production, especially for the materials and equipment produced for the war [4, 5]. The Statistical Quality Control system helped factories maintain quality with mass production [23]. These techniques became very popular in the United States at that time. Those statistical tools and control charts provided by Shewhart are being used even nowadays [24, 25].

1.4 Quality Assurance (1950–1970)/Total Quality Management

Shewhart's work was seminal in quality assurance and management. Following Shewhart's work, William Edwards Deming devoted his work to understanding the philosophy of management, quality management, and understanding variation and systematic problem solving [20, 26]. Deming was an engineer and worked as a statistician in the US Agriculture Department and Census Bureau. He went to Japan in 1945 and was instrumental in using the concept of quality management in Japanese industries to help revive the Japanese economy following World War II setbacks [27, 28]. After World War II, there was a surge in making quality products in Japan [4, 5]. Deming followed the Statistical Quality Control system developed by Shewhart and his management and problem-solving theories to help transform Japan's production processes.

Another name in quality management is Joseph Juran [16], who is remembered as the pioneer of many quality management initiatives. He was another American invited to Japan for collaboration and coordination to uplift the Japanese economy besides Deming. Juran emphasized the importance of human factors, such as leaders and managers, and did not limit quality management to planning, controlling, and improving products [20, 29]. Because of these individuals' insights, Japan opened to cooperation and collaboration with other countries and diverted its production focus from military arms and equipment to quality household products. Japanese focused on overall quality improvement by improving the whole organizational procedure involved in the development of products, moving toward the assurance procedure (Quality Assurance). They introduced Company Wide Quality Control (CWQC) in 1960 instead of statistical quality control [30]. In 1969, the Japanese first-time presented TQM's concept (Total Quality Management) in an International quality management conference [16, 19]. The TQM applied to the management of quality of work of all employees ranging from workers to the head of a particular organization [31]. The United States was still focused on Quality Control through the inspection of products and goods at the end of the manufacturing procedure and removing the defective lots. Later, the United States embraced and embarked upon adopting the Total Quality Management Approach.

1.5 International Organization for Standardization

International Organization for Standardization (ISO) is a special international agency, which developed a series of standards to maintain quality levels at the international level. The organization had 160 countries following the norms developed by the organization. At present, globally, 178 countries have adopted these guidelines, and over 1 million registrations of organizations from various countries have been made [32]. ISO was established in 1987 [16]. Each country has its national standard bodies that participate in ISO and maintain quality in the country based on ISO guidelines; ISO guidelines can be adopted by diverse industries and work areas for maintaining quality [33]. These guidelines are mainly concerned with the documentation of all the processes involved in manufacturing or developing a service or a product.

ISO 9000 is a series developed by ISO to define Quality management and Quality assurance procedures for various companies to follow and maintain overall quality and meet the requirements of industry and companies [34]. The series was first published in March 1987. Later on, it was updated periodically to meet the evolving needs of the markets and businesses (Table 1.1). Along with ISO9000, the ISO developed guidelines for quality management in other fields as well, such as ISO 14000 (Environment management), ISO 26000 (Social responsibility guidelines), and ISO 31000 (Guidelines for management of risks).

Table 1.1 Updated versions of ISO 9000 series. The ISO 9000 series was updated in 2000, 2008, and 2015 after got published in 1987

Sr. no.	ISO updated versions	Year	Goals and principles to achieve
1.	ISO9000:1994	1994	More focus was on preventive actions to improve quality. Emphasized Quality Assurance.
1.	ISO 9000:2000	2000	Five goals were laid to achieve. It should meet the needs of stakeholders. It should be simple enough to understand and implement. It should apply to various sectors. It should apply to all organizations despite their size. It should connect quality systems and business processes [34].
2.	ISO 9000:2008	2008	Documentation. Management commitment. Customer satisfaction. Corrective measures. Training of personnel and management of resources. Planning and design. Process control. Analysis of process. Continuous improvement [35].
3.	ISO 9000:2015 (Latest version)	2015	Seven management principles were there. Continuous improvement in processes and performance. Decisions should be evidence based. Consumer and users should be satisfied. Relationships and collaborations should be well maintained. Process approach. Engagement of people. Leadership [34, 36].

Note: Organization following ISO 9000 are certified for following these norms as ISO 9001 certified

1.6 Great Failures of Quality

Failures of quality management make an important part of the history of Quality assurance. Despite having various quality assurance measures, some of the failures present the importance of quality and rigorous actions that need to be followed to prevent such historical failures of quality. Table 1.2 represents such events; all these organizations were ISO and Q.S. certified [37].

Table 1.2 Failures of quality. Failures of the past's quality management in various organizations caused colossal damage and could have been very dangerous for humankind

Sr. No.	Organization	Year	Failure	Associated casualties
1.	Ford	Since 2004	Recall of over 24 million vehicles for malfunction	No casualty reported
2.	Honda	2011	Recall of 1 million vehicles because of electrical problems	No casualty reported
3.	Endo Pharmaceuticals	NA	Recall of 1.4 million packages of birth control pills because of labelling error in the sequence of taking the pills	No casualty reported
4.	Mattel	2007	Recalled over 11 million toys because of the danger of lead paint and small magnets that could cause choking hazards	No casualty reported
5.	Bridgestone/ Firestone tires	1994, 2000	Recalled over six million tyres	46 deaths

1.7 Good Manufacturing Practices, Good Clinical Practices, and Good Laboratory Practices

Quality assurance is a field that has developed over the years and permeated into various sectors to ensure the quality of work. Various guidelines and practices have been put forth to achieve the goal of quality assurance. According to the field of work, there are three main domains that provide regulations and guidelines for maintaining quality in an organization.

1.7.1 Good Manufacturing Practices

For manufacturing companies, these guidelines are provided under the name of Good Manufacturing Practices (GMP). The first proposal of GMP was finalized in 1963 [38, 39]. Regulation in the manufacture of pharmaceuticals and food products became indispensable because of various past events in the manufacture of drugs, medical devices, and food supplements that could have caused hazards. Table 1.3 enlists some of such events that made it essential to maintain quality in such companies. FDA originated in 1906 after the book "the jungle" was published, which exposed various such events. In 1938 Food Drug and Cosmetic Act was passed [40]. The final rule for GMP was published in 1978 for drugs and medical devices [38, 41].

1.7.2 Good Clinical Practices

For practices in hospitals and clinics, quality management guidelines were named Good Clinical Practices (GCP). GCP also lays down the guidelines and regulations for conducting clinical trials for various drugs. Q.A. (quality assurance) personnel

Table 1.3 Events that prompted companies to maintain quality

Sr. no.	Year	Events
1.	1905	The Jungle Book
2.	1933	America's Chamber of Horrors
3.	1935	Elixir of Sulfanilamide
4.	1944	Public Health Services Act
5.	1941, 1945	Lot wise testing and approval by the FDA (insulin, penicillin, respectively)
6.	1955	Failure to inactivate the poliovirus
7.	1960	Thalidomide tragedy
8.	1982	Poisoned Acetaminophen capsules
9.	1983	Requirements for batch certification were dropped

have important roles in clinical trials for establishing the effectiveness and safety of a drug or procedure. Along with malpractice in the manufacture of drugs and food products, the clinical trials for new drug approval were also being practised in an ill-defined manner. Unethical practices by medical researchers were not uncommon, and participants' safety and well-being were ignored. To prevent malpractice, the Nuremberg Code was established following the infamous Nazi's trial [42, 43]. In 1964, the World Medical Association proposed a formal and more stringent statement than the Nuremberg code known as the Declaration of Helsinki [44, 45]. The Helsinki declaration reinforced the health of patients having precedence over every other aspect of research. The latest update in this declaration was brought in 2008 [46]. During the 1970s and 1980s, different worldwide guidelines were being practised, which impacted pharmaceutical manufacturers' efficacy and efficiency worldwide. The International Conference on Harmonisation of Good Clinical Practice (ICH-GCP) came into existence to address these problems. Nowadays, these guidelines are being practised for clinical trials on human subjects.

1.7.3 Good Laboratory Practice

In 1972, in order to maintain quality in nonclinical practices (pertaining to environmental health, safety, and processes involved in clinical studies), to regulate activities involving toxicity and hazards in chemical laboratories, and to systematize and standardize research planning, execution, monitoring, recording, and reporting, Good Laboratory Practices (GLP) for quality and verifiability purposes were introduced [47]. Term GLP was first time introduced in New Zealand and Denmark [48, 49]. The aim of GLP guidelines was quality assurance in clinical research. The origin of GLP in the United States originated following the incidence of Industrial Bio-Test Inc., which posed a doubt of integrity for more than 200 pesticides associated with inaccurate reports and obscure data [50]. In 1970, four scientists faced a trial, and the company, Industrial Bio-Test Inc. (IBT), Illinois, USA, was alleged for giving false reports of around 200 chemicals [37]. Considering the harmful effects of pesticides on the environment, the 1970's Environmental Protection Act (EPA) was formed in the United States to test the safety of pesticides [51]. That was the reason in the early 1970s, nearly 40 toxicology laboratories were tested for the quality of the research along with IBT. Other companies and laboratories were also found providing fraudulent data regarding the chemicals and pesticides being tested in these laboratories. Similar to the IBT case, the other major fraudulent data was presented by G.D. Searle & Company of Illinois [52, 53]; the company was involved in the production of drugs and food products named Flagyl, Aldactone, and Aspartame. Flagyl was later on found to be tumorigenic for animals. Aldactone was also found to have carcinogenic effects. These events were the marker of unregulated malpractices and a need to regulate nonclinical practices, environmental safety, documentation, reporting, and achieving using good laboratory practices. GLP was first published in the United States in 1978 and became law in 1979 [52]. Some changes were made in 1984, and the final rule was published in 1987. GLP lays down the guidelines for maintaining quality in the practices involved in nonclinical activities, production, and testing the toxicity of various chemicals. The GLP guidelines were adopted by OECD (Organisation for Economic Cooperation and Development) in 1992 [54].

All these efforts were directed toward improving the quality of research in laboratories. Preservation of resources and animals involved in testing and the use of chemicals became a big issue due to the burgeoning list of chemicals used in laboratories and industries [55]. To prevent overuse of resources and animals and improve the quality of data produced by various laboratories, the OECD published new guidelines in 1981 [56, 57]. According to these guidelines, the data for the toxicity of a chemical produced by an OECD member country will be accepted in all other countries. There is no need to duplicate data in other countries. This agreement is known as Mutual Acceptance of Data (MAD). In 1997, non-OECD countries also accepted the policies of MAD [54].

1.8 Origin of GLP in India

In India, the GLP was first introduced in 1983 [58], following GLP and OECD principles. The first usage of insecticides in India took place in 1948 in the form of DDT for malaria control and then for locusts. Without having a standardized procedure, the insecticides were used inconsistently and without considering the ill effects that they may cause on the environment. Many people died in the state of Tamilnadu, India, in 1958. As a result, the Insecticides Act of 1968 was published. Later in 1980, the National Coordination of Testing and Calibration Facilities (NCTCF) was set up by DST (Department of Science and Technology) of Govt. of India. In 1990, the NCTCF was converted to NABL (National Accreditation Board for Testing and Calibration Laboratories), a constituent board of Quality Council of India. NABL follows ISO guidelines and helps in the accreditation of Indian laboratories to international norms [48]. Also, NABL provides accreditation to laboratories for testing and approving chemicals and pesticides in India [49].

Along with NABL, NGCMA (National GLP Compliance Monitoring Authority) is established in India for the maintenance of the quality of nonclinical health and safety data/studies of GLP laboratories, as certification is voluntary. National GLP Compliance Monitoring Authority was established by DST in 2002, and India became a member of OECD in 2011, agreeing to the norms of Mutual Acceptance of Data (MAD). India was the third emerging economy or developing country to become a MAD member after Singapore and South Africa [58].

1.9 Quality Council of India

In 1997, the Quality Council of India (QCI) was established to safeguard users' best interest in various services and products in India [59, 60]. QCI came into existence to provide attestation and accreditation to organizations and companies involved in various trades, such as health care, toxicity, and pharma laboratories, industries, in the area of education and training. The main aim of the QCI is to preserve quality. QCI is a National Quality Campaign which was started with a tagline "Creating an ecosystem for Quality" by the Department of Industrial Policy and Promotion (DIPP) under the Ministry of Commerce and Industry [59]. The concept of QCI first came in 1992 when a need for an accreditation body was realized for industries along with laboratories. In 1996 the idea was proposed in the cabinet, and the Quality Council of India was established in 1997 [61]. Three other prominent organizations coordinated with QCI: Associated Chambers of Commerce and Industry in India (ASSOCHAM), Federation of Indian Chambers of Commerce and Industry (FICCI), and Confederation of Indian Industry (CII) [60]. QCI is made of four components, the lower one being the Accreditation boards and the upper one being the Governing Council [37]. The Accreditation boards consist of NABCB (National Accreditation Board for Certification Bodies), NABET (National Accreditation Board for Education and Training), NABL (National Accreditation for Testing and Calibration Laboratories), and NABH (National Accreditation for Hospitals and Healthcare Providers). NABCB grants accreditation to organizations in areas such as environmental management, information security, and food safety. NABET provides accreditation to education/training institutes and facilities for students, NABL to laboratories involved in testing and calibrations, and NABH to hospitals, clinics, AYUSH (Ayurveda, Yoga & Naturopathy, Unani, Siddha, Sowa-Rigpa, and Homoeopathy) centers, and other such centers concerned with the health sector [62].

The history of Quality Assurance and the various efforts made to maintain quality provide a firm foundation for furthering quality management and good quality management practices. However, the Quality Assurance and GLP system are yet to be utilized effectively in academia and research laboratories. There is a compelling need for implementing quality and GLP systems to increase accountability in research laboratories and enhance the quality of research, efficacy, and reproducibility of results.

This book aims to help all stakeholders who want to benefit from adopting and establishing a GLP system. The upcoming chapters explain in detail the various aspects and requirements for embracing and establishing the GLP system. The GLP system's principal provision is data integrity, verifiability, procedural credibility, and accountability. Research data audit ensures the authenticity and efficacy of the outcomes.

The concept of the audit comes from the need for accounting. Knowledge of audit has been mentioned in the ancient texts of Kautilya named Arthashastra. Arthashastra emphasized personal duty and upheld the righteousness of behavior, conduct, and attitude in economic pursuits for the greater good. In India, the Institute for charter accountants was established in 1880 to prepare auditors [63]. Earlier, the audit was mainly focused on cash exchange transactions, but its focus shifted in the 1970s to include the system and processes [64]. The process of data auditability has been explained in more detail in the chapter entitled "Conceptual framework for research data auditability." For auditing and maintaining quality, skilled human resources are required, and proper training of all personnel involved in any organization is another important requirement for GLP, which has been explained in the chapter entitled "Management of Skilled Human Resource by the Youth-Oriented Good Laboratory." Also, a trained Q.A. (Quality Assurance) person is needed to assess the quality of production and service being provided by an organization. But even the most skilled persons can commit mistakes if they do not follow some quality guidelines and procedures consistently, which necessitates the requirement to follow standardized protocols with built-in checks and balances. The fourth chapter, entitled "Operationalisation of research SOPs for Ph.D. Scholars," deals with the operationalization of SOPs (Standard Operating Procedures), and modules for making SOPs efficacious, have been described. To assess the effective implementation of the SOPs and their compliance in laboratories or companies, real-time data entry following steps of an SOP and using Data Recording Sheets (DRS) is crucial for quality assurance. The procedure for creating DRS has been explained in the chapter, creating data recording sheet (DRS) in the quality management system. While performing any work or generating any data, it is essential to note all the steps and procedures followed in a sheet to enhance the data's integrity and the experiments' reproducibility.

Decreasing productivity loss and maintaining efficiency have always been daunting tasks in academia. Maintaining productivity and keeping the personnel motivated, a proper plan, and its implementation are prerequisites. A good work plan with clear expectations, realistic timelines, crisis management steps, procedural steps to manage external variables, distractions, services, and ethical guidelines can improve productivity, work environment, and information flow. Such measures can contribute to solidifying further accountability in human and other resource management. There is an important parameter in the GLP system to define a timeline for the whole month's work, and it is mandatory to follow the timeline. There can also be a self-proposed timeline that individuals can make themselves for their own benefit and enhance productivity. This timeline is named as Master schedule (MS) in the GLP system. The chapter entitled "The value of Master Schedules in benchmarking research productivity" has elaborated in detail on the value of MS.

As defined earlier, the book's main aim is to present a guide for those who want to establish the GLP system in their laboratories, mainly for research and academic laboratories. The following chapters present systematic guidelines for research scholars and professionals working in academia to manage quality, increase productivity, enhance accountability, improve information flow, and secure the integrity of data and outcomes.

Record keeping of the work performed and protocol followed, along with keeping records of the resources used, is equally crucial and challenging. Effective record-keeping practices of resources can help track chemical consumption, their expiry dates, timely and/or effective use of chemicals, and the efficiency of the chemical or instrument's performance. Keeping log sheet records of chemical scan contribute positively to financial sustainability and waste management. Log sheets are mainly of two types: laboratory and personal. Personal log sheets are required to maintain records of research scholars' academic progress, whereas laboratory log sheets track the laboratories's resources, information, and internal transactions. The log sheets can help fulfil the legal requirements, obligations, and be instrumental in applying for a patent, avoiding inventorship issues. Log sheets can help scholars in keeping track of progress, which is explained in the chapter.

As described earlier, Quality Assurance is an indispensable part of the quality management system. Quality assurance must be implemented by trained personnel who is a Q.A. person and can invigilate any kind of misconduct in research or resource management issues. The focus of the book is to enhance accountability, improve human and material resources management, avert allegations of misconduct, data fraud, and fulfil financial and ethical obligations. The chapter dealing with data fraud (Data fraud and essence of data verifiability) describes the various kinds of data fraud carried out in the past. The historical overview in this chapter can help enhance people's understanding of data frauds jeopardizing the lives of many. Data verifiability has become an integral part of the quality management system and the GLP system to provide high-quality data and prevent data fraud in laboratories. The chapter details the various falsification and plagiarism reports with case reports. Institutional mechanisms and penalties have also been described. Documents handling and record management have been emphasized and mentioned with clear steps. The preserved documents, data, and records can help provide the traceability of fraudulent data. As a result, the archiving of documents in a proper fashion is essential and has been explained in the chapter. The role of document control and archiving records in management, along with data fraud, the lack of quality regulations can generate academic and ethical conflicts as well. Without proper records, false allegations of data fraud can tarnish scientists' credibility and generate inventorship conflicts. How can these academic conflicts be avoided has been presented in the chapter "Instigation and Adherence to the Quality Assurance Programme to Avoid Academic Conflicts." Various orientation models have been discussed in the chapters to keep the staff and scholars motivated and conflict-free. Laboratory orientations are also entrusted to maintain the safety of the staff and the laboratory.

All the persons working in a chemical laboratory need to be familiar with the MSDS (Material Safety Data Sheet) of all chemicals placed in these areas along with the first aid facilities. Such orientation procedures have been explained in the chapter, laboratory orientations, meetings, and value of communication. Communication is vital for maintaining a healthy environment, and it can be enhanced through two interfaces: regular meetings and the activities related to Academic Social Responsibility (ASR). Academic Social responsibility has been made compulsory by DST (Department of Science and Technology) in India. Also, this is ethically pertinent that science institutes connect with communities and understand their social responsibility. ASR is a part of the quality assurance system and is discussed in the chapter "Academic Social Responsibility and Quality Assurance in the Developing World."

Overall, this entire effort, the GLP system, and quality management have become complementary to maintain the quality and high level of service and research, ensuring the well-being of staff and researchers while contributing to society's well-being in general. Different models and approaches to research data generation and consumption have been highlighted in all the book chapters. Maintaining data quality is as essential as the generation of data. The data integrity can be maintained by digitizing the records and documents. Paper archiving is equally important, and it has its associated risks of losing data over time. Preserving data and records in a digitized format can minimize such risks. Technological advancements have made it possible to preserve and protect large datasets while maintaining data integrity. The last chapter, "The Impact of Data Digitization on Data Integrity" describes the procedure of digitization and the nature of digitized data with the help of various software. The book covers the entire cycle of quality in a system and how to integrate it into research, academic, or institutional level with specific details of implementation procedures of Quality Assurance.

References

1. Greenhill S. The changing patterns of work satisfaction. Can Med Assoc J. 1958 Feb 15;78(4):266.
2. Rosser G. Crafts, guilds and the negotiation of work in the medieval town. Past Present. 1997 Feb;1(154):3–1.
3. Young HH. A brief history of quality assurance and peer review. Prof Psychol. 1982 Feb;13(1):9.
4. Berwick DM. Controlling variation in health care: a consultation from Walter Shewhart. Med Care. 1991 Dec;1:1212–25.
5. Marsh P. The new industrial revolution: consumers, globalisation and the end of mass production. New Haven: Yale University Press; 2012 Jul 17.
6. Knegt R. Labour constitutions and market logics: a socio-historical approach. Soc Leg Stud. 2018 Aug;27(4):512–28.
7. Cesaretti R, Lobo J, Bettencourt LM, Ortman SG, Smith ME. Population-area relationship for medieval European cities. PLoS One. 2016 Oct 5;11(10):e0162678.
8. Epstein SA. Wage labor and guilds in medieval Europe. Chapel Hill: UNC Press Books; 1991.
9. Ogilvie S. The economics of guilds. J Econ Perspect. 2014 Nov;28(4):169–92.
10. Humphreys GH. Guild medicine. Ann Surg. 1950 Oct;132(4):844.
11. Tulchinsky TH, Varavikova EA. A history of public health. In: The New Public Health, vol. 1. New York: Elsevier; 2014.
12. Brooks FW. William de Wrotham and the Office of Keeper of the King's Ports and Galleys. English Hist Rev. 1925 Oct 1;40(160):570–9.

13. Brooks DH. Physicians and the pressures of industrialisation. Am J Public Health. 1975 Feb;65(2):182–3.
14. Uddin N, Hossain F. Evolution of modern management through taylorism: an adjustment of scientific management comprising behavioral science. Proc Comput Sci. 2015 Jan 1;62:578–84.
15. Taylor FW, Taylor FW. The father of scientific management. FB Coley Edited. 1923;2
16. Hamid SR, Isa S, Chew BC, Altun A. Quality management evolution from the past to present: challenges for tomorrow. Organizacija. 2019 Aug 1;52(3):157–86.
17. Copley FB, Taylor FW. Father of scientific management. New York: Harper and Brothers; 1923.
18. Chambers JW, Carosso VP. The tyranny of change: America in the progressive era, 1900-1917. New York: St. Martin's Press; 1980.
19. Shewhart WA, Deming WE. Statistical method from the viewpoint of quality control. North Chelmsford: Courier Corporation; 1986.
20. Best M, Neuhauser D. Walter A Shewhart, 1924, and the Hawthorne factory. Qual Saf Health Care. 2006 Apr 1;15(2):142–3.
21. Walter BD, Shewhart A. Economic control of quality of manufactured product (1931). In: Landmark writings in Western mathematics 1640-1940. New York: Elsevier; 2005 Jan 1. p. 926–35.
22. Franco BC, Celano G, Castagliola P, Costa AF. Economic design of Shewhart control charts for monitoring autocorrelated data with skip sampling strategies. Int J Prod Econ. 2014 May 1;151:121–30.
23. American Society for Quality (ASQ). Quality Assurance and Quality Control [Internet]. https://asq.org/quality-resources/quality-assurance-vs-control. Accessed 1 Dec 2020
24. Human SW, Chakraborti S, Smit CF. Shewhart-type control charts for variation in phase I data analysis. Comput Stat Data Anal. 2010 Apr 1;54(4):863–74.
25. Celano G, Castagliola P, Chakraborti S. Joint Shewhart control charts for location and scale monitoring in finite horizon processes. Comput Ind Eng. 2016 Nov 1;101:427–39.
26. Deming WE. Out of the crisis. Cambridge, MA: MIT Press; 2018 Oct 16.
27. Johnson BE. In the library: deming management at work. Strategic Finance. 1992 Feb 1;73(8):14.
28. Tsutsui WM. W. Edwards Deming and the origins of quality control in Japan. J Jpn Stud. 1996 July 1;22(2):295–325.
29. Gryna FM, Juran JM. Quality planning and analysis: from product development through use. New York: McGraw-Hill; 2001.
30. Peterson R, Barker M. Company wide quality control in Japan: implications for Western management practices. Policy Org Soc. 1992 June 1;4(1):83–91.
31. Kiran DR. Total quality management: key concepts and case studies. Oxford: Butterworth-Heinemann; 2016 Oct 28.
32. 9000Store. ISO 9000 series of Quality Standards [Internet]. Available from https://the9000store.com/what-are-iso-9000-standards/. Accessed 1 Dec 2020
33. Kent R. Quality management in plastics processing. New York: Elsevier; 2016 Nov. p. 30.
34. American Society for Quality (ASQ). What is the ISO9000 Standards series [Internet]. https://asq.org/quality-resources/iso-9000. Accessed 1 Dec 2020.
35. 9000Store. ISO 9001:2008 Requirements in plain English [Internet]. https://the9000store.com/iso-9000-tips-iso-9001-requirements/. Accessed 1 Dec 2020.
36. Jasiulewicz-Kaczmarek M. ISO 9000: 2015 quality management principles as the framework for a maintenance management system. Zeszyty Naukowe Politechniki Poznańskiej. Organizacja i Zarządzanie. 2016(69):49–65.
37. Schneider K. Faking it: the case against industrial bio-test laboratories. Amicus J. 1983;1983:14–26.
38. Shukla J. Good Manufacturing Practice (GMP): an overview.
39. U.S. Food and Drug Administration. Good Manufacturing Practices for the 21st century for food processing (2004 study) section 1: Current Food Good Manufacturing Practices[Internet]. 2004; Updated27 Dec 2017. https://www.fda.gov/food/current-good-manufacturing-practices-

cgmps-food-and-dietary-supplements/good-manufacturing-practices-21st-century-food-processing-2004-study-section-1-current-food-good. Accessed 1 Dec 2020.
40. Jain SK, Jain RK. Evolution of GMP in pharmaceutical industry. Res J Pharm Technol. 2017;10(2):601–6.
41. Immel BK. A brief history of the GMPs for pharmaceuticals. Pharm Technol. 2001 Jul;25(7):44–53.
42. Vijayananthan A, Nawawi O. The importance of good clinical practice guidelines and its role in clinical trials. Biomed Imaging Interven J. 2008 Jan;4(1):e5.
43. Williams JR. The Declaration of Helsinki and public health. Bull World Health Organ. 2008;86:650–2.
44. Carlson RV, Boyd KM, Webb DJ. The revision of the Declaration of Helsinki: past, present and future. Br J Clin Pharmacol. 2004 Jun;57(6):695–713.
45. Malik AY, Foster C. The revised Declaration of Helsinki: cosmetic or real change? J R Soc Med. 2016 May;109(5):184–9.
46. Garrafa V, Lorenzo C. Moral imperialism and multi-centric clinical trials in peripheral countries. Cad Saude Publica. 2008 Oct;24(10):2219–26.
47. World Health Organization. Handbook: good laboratory practice (GLP): quality practices for regulated non-clinical research and development. World Health Organization; 2010 Feb 2.
48. Shukla S, Shankar R, Singh SP. Food safety regulatory model in India. Food Control. 2014 Mar 1;37:401–13.
49. Sitaraman R. Incorporating good laboratory practices in academic research laboratories: prospects and perspectives. In: Proceedings of the National Conference on "GLP and ISO/IEC-17025 - Emphasis on Regulatory Affairs and Application in Academic Research". Chennai: IIBAT. p. 83.
50. Marshall E. The murky world of toxicity testing. Science. 1983;220:1130–2.
51. United States Environmental Protection Agency. Quality assurance guidance document-model quality assurance project plan for the PM ambient air. 2001;2.
52. Baldeshwiler AM. History of FDA good laboratory practices. Qual Assur J. 2003 Sep;7(3):157–61.
53. Smith RJ. Creative penmanship in animal testing prompts FDA controls. Science. 1977;198:1227–9.
54. Kendall G, Bai R, Błazewicz J, De Causmaecker P, Gendreau M, John R, Li J, McCollum B, Pesch E, Qu R, Sabar N. Good laboratory practice for optimisation research. J Oper Res Soc. 2016 Apr 1;67(4):676–89.
55. Becker RA, Janus ER, White RD, Kruszewski FH, Brackett RE. Good laboratory practices and safety assessments. Environ Health Perspect. 2009 Nov;117(11):A482–3.
56. Salzman J. Decentralized administrative law in the Organization for Economic Cooperation and Development. Law Contemp Prob. 2004;68:189.
57. Wollin KM, Harston S, Lilienblum W. Quality assurance in toxicology. Regul Toxicol. 2020;2020:1–9.
58. Rasmussen K, Rauscher H, Kearns P, González M, Sintes JR. Developing OECD test guidelines for regulatory testing of nanomaterials to ensure mutual acceptance of test data. Regul Toxicol Pharmacol. 2019 Jun 1;104:74–83.
59. Nischal PM. Parliamentary committee report on the functioning of Medical Council of India. Natl Med J India. 2016 May 1;29(3):185.
60. Kochanek SA. The transformation of interest politics in India. Pac Aff. 1995 Dec;1:529–50.
61. Khan F, Khan H. Quality management in the healthcare industry. Decision. 2004 July 1;31(2):0304.
62. Hajare P. Quality Council of India [Internet]. 18 Aug 2020. https://pscnotes.in/quality-council-of-india/. Accessed 1 Dec 2020.
63. Verma S, Gray SJ. The creation of the Institute of Chartered Accountants of India: the first steps in the development of an indigenous accounting profession post-independence. Acc Historians J. 2006 Dec;33(2):131–56.
64. Teck-Heang LE, Ali AM. The evolution of auditing: an analysis of the historical development. J Mod Account Audit. 2008 Dec 1;4(12):1.

Conceptual Framework of Research Data Auditability

2

Rahul Tyagi and Venkatesh Thuppil

2.1 Introduction

The World Health Organization (WHO) defines Research as "development of knowledge with the aim of understanding health challenges and mounting an improved response to them." The five major areas being covered in research include "measuring the problem; understanding its cause(s), elaborating solutions; translating the solutions or evidence into policy, practice and products and evaluating the effectiveness of the solutions" [1]. Even though the core principles of basic research were framed on the moral ground initially, the criticality and dimension of research data auditability, has been realized lately. US Food and Drug Administration (FDA) introduced the Good Lab Practices (GLP) in 1976 for the nonclinical studies. Thereafter, the Organisation for Economic Co-operation and Development (OECD) constituted the Good Lab Practices (GLP) under the special program on the control of chemicals in 1978.

Across the globe in the recent COVID-19 global pandemic, the **C**linical **R**esearch **D**ata **M**anagement **(CRDM)** is finding a significant role in the outcome and application of modern-day reliable clinical data in almost all areas of clinical research with special reference to demographic data and data concerning drug trials, vaccine efficacy, and diagnostic requirements. Reliable scientific data generated through various means by systematic and planned clinical research are

R. Tyagi
Neuroscience Research Lab, Department of Neurology, Postgraduate Institute of Medical Education and Research, Chandigarh, Chandigarh, India

Allergy and Immunology Unit, Department of Paediatrics, Advanced Paediatric Centre, Postgraduate Institute of Medical Education and Research, Chandigarh, Chandigarh, India

V. Thuppil (✉)
Department of Biochemistry, St. John's Medical College, Bengaluru, India
e-mail: Venkatesh.thuppil@gmail.com

A. Anand (ed.), *Quality Assurance Implementation in Research Labs*,
https://doi.org/10.1007/978-981-16-3074-3_2

unconditionally accepted. When validated methodology is used to get similar data at a different clinical setup, it is widely accepted by the scientific community. Such data eventually becomes dependable and reproducible across similar researchers working in different locations, provided that their basic resources are comparable. Modern-day clinical researchers have realized that the management of clinical research data, when unconditionally accepted, needs to be sustainable and used for a long period by any researcher to further invent and innovate, using the generated research data. In this context, both basic and applied clinical research is important which includes primarily discovery, invention, and innovations. Discovery refers to what has already existed but not realized till it was found either by systematic and planned study or by mere accidental discovery during clinical studies comprising explorations and investigations. The information gained from what is discovered is subjected to further in-depth probing by the same or different researchers/subject experts. Such information and data often result in inventions using certain intrinsic properties of what is discovered. To make it simple, for example, when an element or virus is discovered, many things are invented using this discovery during the course of time. The invention is further modified and made economically available and scientifically acceptable by many through further innovation.

What is not there cannot be seen or found

True researchers have accepted that they have moved from the classical and traditional methods of generation of new data, which is subsequently presented in scientific meetings leading to an in-depth debate, arguments, and discussions by subject experts. This is apart from presenting the data at annual conferences. However, researchers have realized that in the present day, data management also involves what is more popularly known as conceptual framework. Other means such as publishing the data through peer-reviewed journal articles or quoting in standard textbooks and preparing research reviews, still remain questionable by many for authenticity of the research data as several journals and textbooks lack credibility of their status.

Conceptual framework for clinical research data refers to "the way scientific ideas originated in the minds of researchers in clinical setup, which are systematically organized and planned to achieve what is preconceived in the minds of clinical researchers apart from meeting the research project's purpose as an expected outcome." Conceptual framework is always linked to the main purpose and definite aim of the research. Purpose and aim in this context composed of predictions and various pre-planned means of realizing what is predicted.

A true clinical researcher always dreams of reliable data and chases the dream which keeps the researcher awake till the dream is realized.

Conceptual and theoretical framework for **C**linical **R**esearch **D**ata **M**anagement **(CRDM)** involves primarily identifying the variables that have significant influences on the research data generated, apart from mapping the interaction of these variables and understanding how they can have an impact on the research data used for decision-making. Sharing of the research data through open access publications eventually helps in promoting the growth of research and development and reduces duplication of hard work. Conceptual and theoretical frameworks are distinctly similar; a few differences have been outlined below.

Conceptual framework: The key to the conceptual framework is strong literature support, which develops after rigorous literature review. The hypothesis associated with the framework is then tested. Sometimes, conceptual framework is redefined, refined to meet the personalized research model or research framework.

Theoretical framework normally adheres to theories, models, and frameworks that one has to review during a literature survey. Normally, a researcher will develop their conceptual framework based on previous theoretical designs. Theoretical frameworks are important, as without them a conceptual framework may not work.

The visual format of the conceptual framework for research data makes its management more effective and saves time and resources. Variables that influence the research data management need to be correlated in the visual framework. This is normally done by adopting any or all of the following by constructing the conceptual framework by:

- *Firstly, identifying the significant key performance variables (KPV) which are commonly used in the specific performance area (SPA) of the research study outcome.*
- *To prepare key performance variables within what is realized about the subject area which primarily covers both current and earlier review of published literature.*
- *Finally, segregating them as either dependent or independent key performance/specific variables in the management of research data.*

However, the conceptual framework is a powerful analytical tool that is used to get a comprehensive understanding of a research concept/phenomenon during data generation. A conceptual framework always helps the researchers in formulating a plan as to what to expect and find through their research, whether their intent of research through appropriate data management is realized or not. Methods employed in empirical research are concerned with verifiable observations rather than mere theory, or even pure logic which can provide a greater insight into research data management *"they provided considerable empirical evidence to support their argument."*

Research data auditability is a basic requirement to ensure the quality and adequacy of research data. A planned and systematic research data generating system is often referred to as Quality Management System (QMS), which needs to be validated by the researchers/research team involved through an independent audit of the system and the outcome has to be verified using audit tools by any independent party competent to audit the system. This can be easily achieved by checking well-kept records, transparency of its operational reporting, provided the managers provide substantial paperwork to the **auditor**. The audit involves checking the structural requirements, the processes adopted, and finally the reliability of outcome of the data. When a similar audit process is done by an independent third-party audit, it results in accreditation.

2.2 Clinical Research Data Management (CRDM) and Conceptual Framework and QRMS

As we had earlier noted, the scientific ideas that originated in the minds of researchers have to result in the expected outcome of research data based on several decisions which require quality resources to be handled by competent people in Clinical Research Organization (CROs). This can happen only where **Q**uality **C**linical **R**esearch **M**anagement **S**ystem **(QCRMS)** is in place.

2.3 Essential Eight Quality Resources for Any Research Organization Are (5M, + 2E, + & 1I)

1. **Manpower in the research organization must be highly competent**. Competency is the combination of appropriate qualification, adequate training, and sufficient experience. However, the combination of competence, righteousness, and courage to speak out the truth results in skills much needed for generating research data.
2. **Management must be committed and passionate about research and the research data**. The management of the research organization has a great role to play apart from having legal entity, responsibility, and commitment. It is appropriate to have management with adequate knowledge about the goals and objectives set by the research organization.
3. **Mechanism/machinery must be foolproof at all times while generating research data**. This refers to the process flow at all levels of work.
4. **Methods used must be validated and verified before use.** This ensures that valid research data be obtained. Validated methods must be subjected to the process of verification provided that no changes in the validated method are made in-house.
5. **Material procured and used in the research process to generate valid data must be of ensured quality.**
6. **Equipment used to quantify and measure must be calibrated by the accredited calibration laboratories and should be well maintained.**
7. **The environment under which the research data is generated must be controlled, monitored, and recorded in addition to being periodically reviewed for its suitability.**
8. **Information management must be reliable. Whatever is applicable to equipment is also applicable to information used in the data management.**

All of the above eight resources form the structural requirements of the research organization are essential to generate research data. The final clinical research data obtained will be the true outcome, which is dependent on the appropriate processes adopted. Hence **Structure-Process-Outcome** based research data is acceptable provided it is based on a **mutually agreed upon standard**. In order to ensure the appropriateness of this requirement, the management needs to have well documented and implementable policies understood by all the clinical researchers. What is understood needs to be implemented by adopting validated procedures and finally, the only evidence that these are truly in place is evidenced and supported by the records. This type of research organizational system is considered as Quality Research Management System (QRMS) [2].

> Quality is never an accident-it is always the result of high intention, sincere effort, intelligent direction and skillful execution; it represents the wise choice of many alternatives—William A Foster

2.4 Importance of Quality Assurance and Quality Control While Looking at Clinical Research Data

2.4.1 Quality Assurance (QA)

*In clinical research is a way of preventing mistakes or defects while generating research data and avoiding problems when delivering solutions or services to end-users of the clinical data; which ISO 9000 defines as **"part of Quality Management System referred above which is focused on providing confidence that quality requirements will be fulfilled."***

"The terms ***"quality assurance"*** and ***"quality control"*** are often used interchangeably to refer to ways of ensuring the quality of a service that uses research data in research organizations. The terms, however, have different meanings. *Assurance:* The act of giving confidence, the state of being certain, or the act of making certain. *Quality Assurance:* The planned and systematic activities implemented in a quality system so that the quality requirements of valid research data will be fulfilled. *Control:* An evaluation to indicate needed corrective responses; the act of guiding a process in which variability is attributable to a constant system of chance causes. *Quality control:* The observation techniques and activities used to fulfill requirements for quality. This is where the measurement of uncertainty in the data generated/obtained will play a major role in providing dependable information based on which decisions can be taken.

Let us consider as an example, the use of appropriate quality control from a medical research perspective:

Quality control is required in clinical research to monitor the performance of the research procedure, to ensure the reliability of data generated, to maintain both precision and accuracy. In many countries, quality control (QC) also means "internal" quality control (IQC).

Controls in medical research are of three types:

(a) Commercial lyophilized material (assayed; the values are known).
(b) Commercial stabilized, low-temperature liquid material (assayed; the values are known).
(c) Pooled serum prepared in-house (unassayed, values not known).

Commercial lyophilized material is reconstituted using laboratory deionized water, as per the procedure provided by the manufacturer/supplier. The low-temperature liquid material eliminates pipetting error as there is no reconstitution step. The in-house pooled serum is prepared by pooling the leftover serum samples provided the measurand is well preserved (Measurand is the property of the analyte which is estimated, based on which the methodology is developed and validated, for which the accreditation by the third party is obtained). The internal quality control samples should test negative for HIV and hepatitis B viruses.

The control measurements are made only after the control materials are dispensed as aliquots in small volumes (about 500 μL) in vials. The control materials should mimic the patients' samples (should have the same matrix characteristics as the patient's sample which includes contents, color, and viscosity). Adopting appropriate quality control has always ensured reliable research data as seen in medical research. This helps in creating conceptual frameworks that are connected to a research purpose or aim at minimizing the uncertainty factor of research data. Uncertainty of the research data is attributed basically to five variables (causing SWIPE) which are:

- **S**tandard used must be of high quality.
- **W**ork procedure adopted should be validated.
- **I**nstrument calibration must have an unbroken chain of traceability.
- **P**ersonnel must be appropriately trained.
- **E**quipment to measure must be calibrated.

The above framework is based on SWIPE. This can minimize the uncertainty factor of the research data ensuring the validity of the research data. This is an example of the conceptual framework which illustrates what is expected through planned research. It encourages in streamlining the relevant variables for the research and maps out the relation of each other. Research data has a chronological life cycle and phases from the creation, to analysis, organization, validation, storage, and sharing influenced by the uncertainty factor. Considering this to some extent helps in research data management. Apart from this data privacy, data security, copyright, and licensing are of utmost importance. In clinical research, the data needs to be protected as the issue of confidentiality is of prime importance. This factor is normally governed by local, regional, or national clinical research-related regulations and statutory requirements of the state policies concerned [3].

Parsons et al. in their article "A conceptual framework for managing very diverse data for complex, interdisciplinary science" have mentioned that the data should be discoverable, open, linked, useful, and safe. According to them the data must be kept at appropriate locations and shall be traceable, openly accessible in system-dependent manner. It shall be interrelated and connected. Most importantly the data shall be protected from being stolen, lose [4].

Audit with reference to ***Conceptual framework for clinical research data.***

In order to adopt and fulfill quality requirement/s, several tools are used to Assess, Quantify, Monitor, and Report (AQMR) on the application of the data generated during clinical research and to study its Impacts. The most common among them is an audit which requires the concerned clinical researchers to have audit ability.

Apart from this, an audit is a systematic, independent, and documented process for obtaining and checking the clinical data generated and evaluating it objectively to determine the extent to which audit criteria are fulfilled as per the requirement of ISO 19011. Audit of the clinical research involves both, individual data tracer and system tracer methodologies. An audit undertaken by the management is considered as an internal audit while the user of the data conducting an audit is considered as an external audit. During the audit of quality, clinical research quality tools are to be looked into. For example, the Cause and Effect diagram (Ishikawa "fish-bone diagram") identifies many possible causes for an effect or problem and sorts ideas into useful categories while generating scientific data. It can help in brainstorming to identify possible causes of a problem and in sorting ideas into useful categories. A **fishbone diagram** is a visual way to look at cause and effect. The problem or effect is displayed at the head or mouth of the fish. This can be seen on YouTube under Fish-bone cause and effect and root cause analysis.

2.4.2 Auditability

Auditability depends upon many factors such as competency of the auditor, independency provided to the auditor, and unbiased implementation of audit process in clinical research comprising of the following:

- Competent auditors must have good knowledge about the QMS of the clinical research organization (CRO) while conducting the periodic audit of the system.
- CRO must comply with statutory and regulatory requirements while implementing standards, guides, and is required to comply with the International/National/Local/institutional requirements.
- Planned audit and the audit process need to be documented.
- Audit must cover all areas of activities and all concerned in the process.
- The outcome of the audit needs to be reviewed by the management and appropriate action should be taken within the acceptable time limit.
- Auditors can support the quality management system by providing inputs.
- All records and related documents generated during the audit must be retained for a pre-defined period.
- Any limitation on the part of CRO, identified during the audit is to be considered as an opportunity for improvement (which was earlier termed as nonconformance). It must be addressed irrespective of the kind or type of resource requirement.

Audit of the QMS generating the ***clinical research data*** is essential for ensuring the quality of the ***Conceptual framework employed*** [5]. **Auditor's ability** is **defined** as the ability to check the accuracy of the data when they check the organizational QMS. **Auditor's ability** can be influenced by a biased auditor not being sufficiently independent of the entity being audited.

2.4.3 Audit Cycle and Quality Improvement

Auditors need to have a well-defined audit plan. What is planned has to be meticulously audited. The outcome of the audit must go through proper checking for any deviations from the implementation of the QMS while generating the research data. After the root cause and CAPA analysis, measurable quality indicators are used as markers of quality improvement. This audit cycle also called Deming cycle is normally repeated annually so that continual improvement is achieved. The schematic representing the audit cycle has been provided in Fig. 2.1.

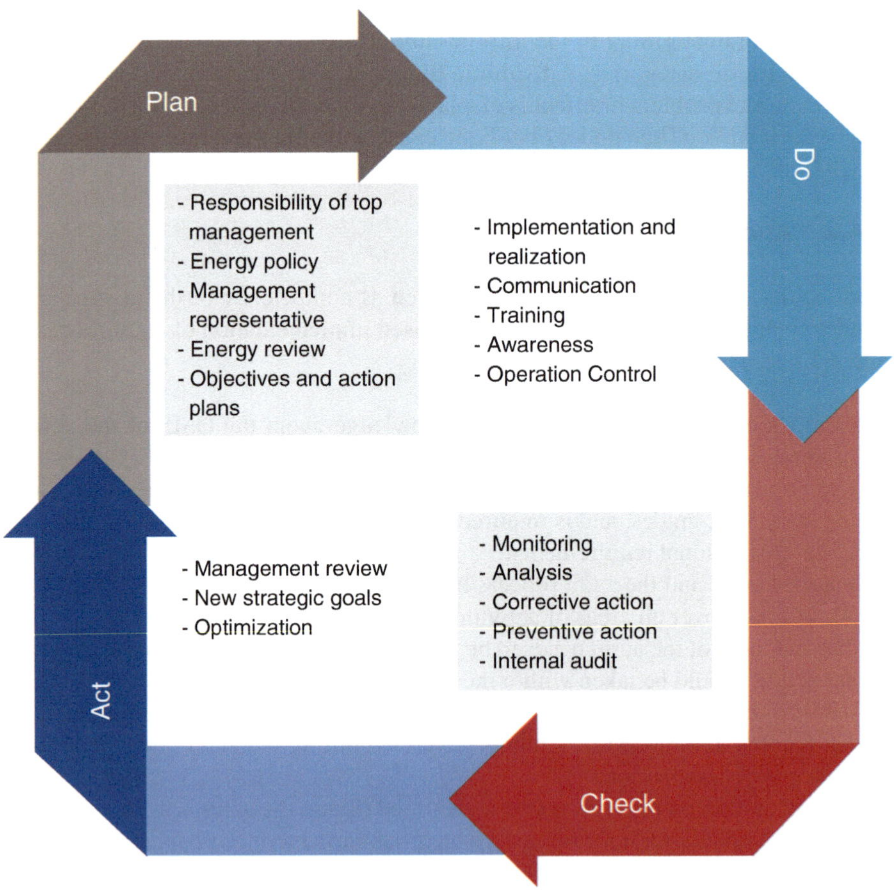

Fig. 2.1 Schematic audit cycle as an example for energy audit [6]

To put it in simple terms, one needs to consider the use of an appropriate conceptual framework to generate dependable, reliable, and verified data, which has to be endorsed during the audit by competent auditors. A planned and documented audit helps in the process of monitoring continual improvement of the entire Quality Management System. Scientific data obtained in clinical research in well-established QMS has to be periodically evaluated through audit. Such a process will be evidenced by improvement in the measurable key performance indicators (KPI).

2.5 Framework for Basic Research Auditing

Basic research has never been included under the purview of quality standards and has resulted in fraudulent reports. Dawson et al. correspondence have published in the *Nature* regarding their concern for initiating the scientific data auditing practise similar to the banking system [7]. Similar suggestions for developing auditable scientific data have also been reported [8–11]. Only a few centers globally could implement the quality research practices in basic research settings.

2.6 Designing the Procedures and Policies for Data Auditing

2.6.1 Preparation of a Quality Manual for Research Laboratory

The objective of preparing a quality manual is to enhance the efficiency, transparency, and accountability of the research facility by establishing a documented quality management system in accordance with international criteria of technical competence. A Quality Manual (QM) should be drafted as a collective effort by all staff including the quality manager and the study director. Personnel having a sound interest in the quality management system such as Good Laboratory Practices (GLP) should be nominated and trained for implementation of the Quality Assurance practices. Research staff should be acquainted with the required documents as well as assessment procedures. QM should clearly define the vision, scope, and objectives of the laboratory along with an organogram of the organization, a structured management system with appropriate rules and regulations, along with mechanisms for advisory services, grievance redressal, purchasing procedures, supplies, service to patients, corrective and preventive actions, document control, Intra-Inter laboratory validations, templates, periodic calibrations, and training. The management shall have responsibility for the design, implementation, maintenance, and improvement of the quality management system for increased transparency, accountability, and efficiency of the diagnostic facility.

QM should be drafted according to the laboratory functioning and vision. Existing scope and objectives in the quality manual should be compared with relevant international and national agencies such as the International Organization for Standardization (ISO) [12], World Health Organization (WHO), Good Laboratory

Practices (GLP) as per the Organisation for Economic Co-operation and Development (OECD), National Accreditation Board for Testing and Calibration Laboratories (NABL), Department of Science and Technology, India (DST), Quality Council of India (QCI), and Bureau of Indian Standards (BIS). QM should be structured to organize the testing laboratories to be compliant and dedicated toward patient care and management with required precision and accuracy. The scope of implementation for clinical testing facilities is stringent as per the government rules. However, the basic research facilities may incorporate overlapping parts from various guidelines for the formulation of the Quality Manual as per laboratory research area and infrastructure.

2.6.2 Personnel

The crucial element in establishing the quality assured facility includes the laboratory personnel or the in Life observer(s). The key responsibilities of the laboratory personnel have been described in Fig. 2.2.

2.6.2.1 Study Director

The study director conceptualizes and plans the activities. He/she is in charge of administrative tasks, financial controls, policy formulations, mobilization, and allocation of human resources and arranging training opportunities to enhance their competence. The Study director ensures that the organization operates smoothly (Fig. 2.2).

2.6.2.2 Quality Assurance and Document Controller

QADC ensures that appropriate standards of quality are followed in the laboratory. Inspections of the facilities, the study, and the infrastructure are held by the QADC. They also prepare, update, and control the quality documents. QADC helps in quality assurance by assisting the study director.

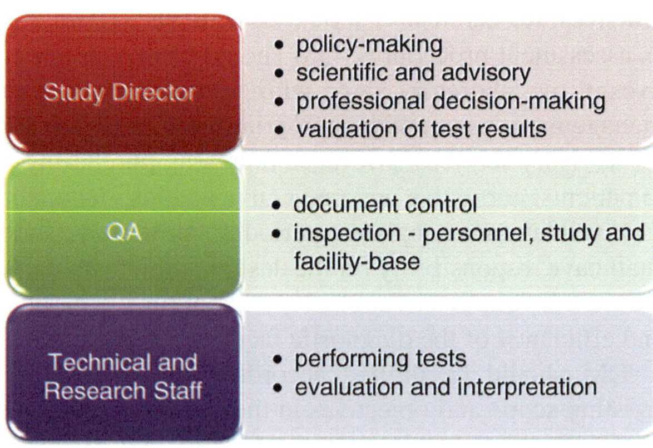

Fig. 2.2 Responsibilities of laboratory personnel

2.6.2.3 Research Staff

The end user of the entire plan may record and maintain the documents pertaining to the individual study.

2.6.2.4 Laboratory Technician

Their responsibility is to perform tests in the laboratory, keep records, and communicate with the researchers and patients.

2.6.2.5 Laboratory Assistant

Their responsibility is to get consent forms filled, coding, maintenance of stocks, and entries.

2.7 Research Design

The most critical aspect is proposing a research question that will answer the hitherto un-attempted areas. The research should create new knowledge in the field or correct previous errors by using appropriate methods. Various areas of research functioning may include diagnostic research like genetic screening of disorders, analysis of risk factors and biomarkers, in vivo studies including animal models of various pathologies, and in vitro manipulation of stem cells [13–19]. Maintaining the biorepository of samples including DNA, RNA (cDNA), plasma, serum, and lymphocytes is another area for which requires an in-depth documentation facility.

The design should outline certain objectives for which standard operating procedures would be derived and documented. Pre-planned contribution policies, authorship plans, and plagiarism, and ethical guidelines should be outlined and competing interests should be identified. It is crucial to document the literature support leading to generation of the hypothesis of study design to reduce unnecessary replication of previously established studies. The research plan should spell out the applicability and future perspectives for the basic or clinical research studies indicating its translational capabilities. Based upon the research plan, the adherence to quality assurance practices shall be proposed, streamlined, prepared, and implemented to monitor and audit the research data.

2.7.1 Conduct of Research

Major challenges for maintaining the research data integrity arises because the basic nature of conducting research is on moral grounds. Hence, a system-dependent documentation approach should be developed by the institutions/laboratories rather than person-dependent procedures. For execution of quality-oriented research data collection, principal investigators should develop formats for each step of research as previously reported [20–22]. It is crucial here to identify various steps for data curation and auditing strategies.

2.7.2 Planning

This is one of the most critical steps. It involves documenting the yearly/quarterly, monthly/weekly planning after consultation with the PI/study director/management to prioritize the experimental workflow. A monthly master schedule (MS) shall be proposed by the researcher and submitted to the personnel handling the quality assurance. Besides tracking the output, preparation of MS provides a focused workflow to the research staff. It also keeps track of consumables, infrastructural requirements, and inventory management.

2.7.3 Standard Operating Procedure

Standard Operating Procedures (SOPs) provide uniformity in the research conduct and help establish system-dependent instructions for staff. There shall be an SOP for all procedures in the research facility including an SOP for SOPs. The standardized procedures related to experimental protocols, administrative and accounting procedures, and academic activities shall have an SOP that is duly approved by the study director/management and submitted to QA. The QA independently monitors if the procedures conducted by the researcher adhere to the approved SOP. Conceptually, an SOP defines stringent steps which may not suit the dynamism of basic research. Hence, as per requirements, SOPs can be revised from time to time.

2.7.4 Data Recording Sheets

Besides conventional raw books, there should be pre-formatted documents for real-time monitoring of the experiments. The format of the Data Recording Sheet (DRS) should be prepared under the supervision of the management and approved by the study director. Preferably, each DRS should be obtained from the QA personnel before conducting experiments. The DRS should record the experimental conditions, flow of experiments, lots of instruments, and the consumables and any deviations should be reported during the experiments. The DRS may be submitted to the QA after review from the study director.

2.8 Identification of Problems

2.8.1 Source of Information for Identification of Problems

1. For every single procedure there shall be an in-built SOP, DRS, and, raw book available. Any experimental procedure performed in the laboratory shall be thoroughly followed by its respective SOP and properly documented in its respective DRS and raw book. Any deviation shall be reported in DRS as well as the raw book, which could be the source of information for identification of problems.

2. For every single instrument there shall be a logbook, instruction sheet, and equipment maintenance file available. Any experimental procedure performed through these instruments in the laboratory shall be thoroughly followed through their respective instruction sheet. Any deviation shall be reported in the logbook as well as instrument maintenance file, which could be the source of information for identification of problems.
3. Cause analysis: Sources of information for identification of problems shall be discussed among the experimenter QA personnel and the management to evaluate the cause of deviation and shall be documented in the respective DRS and equipment maintenance file.

2.9 Corrective Action

There shall be an existing laboratory's policy on corrective action when nonconforming work or departures from policies and procedures in the management system or technical operations are identified. The in Life observer(s) may be responsible for planning, implementing, monitoring, and documenting appropriate corrective action for individual instruments, maintenance, calibration, breakdown, and reporting deviations. The in Life observer(s) shall be solely responsible for individual instruments. The researcher shall be responsible for proper reporting and documentation of procedural/technical errors. The QA personnel shall report this to the management and any deviations or amendments in the protocols shall be finalized after thorough discussion between the experimenter, QA personnel, and the management.

2.9.1 Selection and Implementation of Corrective Actions

It shall be the sole responsibility of the management to select the corrective action according to the type of deviation and it shall be implemented by the experimenter or in Life observer(s). The corrective measure shall be documented respectively and informed to the QA personnel also.

2.9.2 Monitoring of Corrective Actions

Corrective actions shall be monitored through respective log sheets, maintenance sheets, and periodical QA reviews. If the deviation is still not rectified, it shall be documented and immediately reported to the QA personnel and Management.

2.9.3 Additional Audits Where Nonconformities/Departures Cast Doubt

1. Additional audits for instruments shall be performed by periodical calibrations and preventive maintenance.

2. Study-based auditing shall be performed in three layers of inspections: weekly inspection by the in Life observer(s)/experimenter, monthly QA review of study-, infrastructure-, and personnel-based inspections, monthly inspection by the management.

2.10 Capacity Building

Personnel involved in testing, research, and analysis of reports/data shall be appropriately trained, qualified, and duly supervised to conduct the procedure. To achieve sustained efficiency of personnel, periodic training shall be scheduled. Competency of the research staff should be evaluated periodically to assess the skill development and effectiveness of training procedures.

2.11 Future Directions and Clinical Implications

Auditors' ability leads to verification of the authenticity of the data generated in clinical research. Normally in any **C**linical **R**esearch **D**ata **M**anagement **(CRDM), conceptual framework** is systematically organized and planned to achieve what is preconceived in the minds of clinical researchers. In the conceptual framework ideas are normally generated based on evidence in the form of data. Hence, total audit of the clinical research data ensures the appropriateness of the conceptual framework supporting CRDM. Scientific integrity requires a system-dependent quality management procedure. Governments and Institutes should adopt need-based modules for establishing quality management systems in the research settings. The new generation of researchers should learn quality management as a part of their curriculum to inculcate the spirit to maintain scientific integrity.

Acknowledgments We thank Dr. Akshay Anand for his visionary thoughts on compiling this book. First, author thanks Neuroscience Research Lab, Dr. Sadasivan Pillai and Dr. Sudhir Srivastava for encouraging him to gain knowledge on this topic.

References

1. WHO. World Health Organization strategy on research for health. 2012.
2. Śwituła D. The concept of quality in clinical research. Sci Eng Ethics. 2006;12:147–56.
3. White GH. Basics of estimating measurement uncertainty. Clin Biochem Rev. 2008;29(Suppl 1):S53–60.
4. Parsons MAGØ, LeDrew E, et al. A conceptual framework for managing very diverse data for complex, interdisciplinary science. J Inf Sci. 2011;37(6):555–69.
5. Kelly MP, Stewart E, Morgan A, Killoran A, Fischer A, Threlfall A, et al. A conceptual framework for public health: NICE's emerging approach. Public Health. 2009;123(1):e14–20.
6. Plan-Do-Check-Act (PDCA). Conceptdraw.com [Internet]. 2020. Available from https://www.conceptdraw.com/solution-park/management-plan-do-check-act.
7. Dawson N. Ensuring scientific integrity. Nature. 1987;327(6123):550.

8. Resnik DB, Shamoo AE. Fostering research integrity. Account Res. 2017;24(6):367–72.
9. Overbeke AJ. Fraud in fundamental and clinical investigations. The necessity for an independent commission for scientific integrity. Verh K Acad Geneeskd Belg. 2004;66(5–6):343–50. discussion 51-2
10. Dworkin G. Fraud and science. Prog Clin Biol Res. 1983;128:65–74.
11. Weinstein D. Scientific fraud and scientific ethics. Conn Med. 1981;45(10):655–8.
12. ISO 19011: Guidelines for auditing management systems & ISO 15189:2012. Medical laboratories—Requirements for quality and competence. 2012.
13. Sharma NK, Gupta A, Prabhakar S, Singh R, Bhatt AK, Anand A. CC chemokine receptor-3 as new target for age-related macular degeneration. Gene. 2013;523(1):106–11.
14. Anand A, Banik A, Thakur K, Masters CL. The animal models of dementia and Alzheimer's disease for pre-clinical testing and clinical translation. Curr Alzheimer Res. 2012;9(9):1010–29.
15. Goyal K, Koul V, Singh Y, Anand A. Targeted drug delivery to central nervous system (CNS) for the treatment of neurodegenerative disorders: trends and advances. Cent Nerv Syst Agents Med Chem. 2014;14(1):43–59.
16. Sharma NK, Gupta A, Prabhakar S, Singh R, Sharma S, Anand A. Single nucleotide polymorphism and serum levels of VEGFR2 are associated with age related macular degeneration. Curr Neurovasc Res. 2012;9(4):256–65.
17. Tyagi R, Kumar S, Dalal A, Mohammed F, Mohanty M, Anand A. Repurposing pathogenic variants of DMD gene and its isoforms for DMD exon skipping intervention. Curr Genomics. 2019;20(7):519–30.
18. Tyagi R, Aggarwal P, Mohanty M, Dutt V, Anand A. Computational cognitive modeling and validation of Dp140 induced alteration of working memory in Duchenne muscular dystrophy. Sci Rep. 2020;10(1):11989.
19. Tyagi R, Podder V, Arvind H, Mohanty M, Anand A. The role of dystrophin gene mutations in neuropsychological domains of DMD boys: a longitudinal study. Ann Neurosci. 2019;26(3–4):42–9.
20. Tyagi R, Anand A. Development and implementation of ZED-YOG quality module: Niyantrita Madhumeha Bharata skill development initiatives. Ann Neurosci. 2019;26(1):37–44.
21. Manghani K. Quality assurance: importance of systems and standard operating procedures. Perspect Clin Res. 2011;2(1):34–7.
22. Kaushal S, Tyagi R, Banik A, Battu P, Mehra P, Sharma NK, et al. A unique data validation process by internal and external quality assurance system aimed to combat research malpractice. Int J Sci Res. 2019;8(8):5–9.

Management of Skilled Human Resources by Youth-Oriented Good Laboratory Practices (YOG)

3

Sheetal J Gupta and Ajay Kumar Sehgal

3.1 Introduction

The quality of the products or services mainly depends upon the employees which constitute the organization. The workforce is an important resource for improving the quality of work and is the central pillar of any organization. The accelerated pace of development in the modern era demands new skills and skilled human resources. Essentially, in order to follow good laboratory practices, skilled and appropriate human resources are needed. The competency and level of skill of human resources engaged should be customized to fit the requirements of the laboratory. It is important to assess the competency of an individual and then train the individual accordingly, which would in turn help the laboratory in improving its overall performance and quality of service.

Under the current economic conditions, unemployment rates, age of the existing employees, and the pattern in which the older workforce retires certainly affects the youth looking for new jobs. The competition is increasing every day and for that the youth is putting in efforts to hone their skills. Switching over for better prospects is now in the blood of the skilled youth. It is essential to understand the current scenario by analyzing the situation and future changes the industry going to face in order to manage the skilled human resources in a youth-oriented good laboratory.

S. J. Gupta
SVYASA, Bengaluru, India

Neuroscience Research Laboratory, Department of Neurology, PGIMER, Chandigarh, Chandigarh, India

A. K. Sehgal (✉)
Society for Petroleum Laboratory, Ministry of Petroleum & Natural Gas, Noida, Uttar Pradesh, India
e-mail: sehgalak57@gmail.com

A. Anand (ed.), *Quality Assurance Implementation in Research Labs*,
https://doi.org/10.1007/978-981-16-3074-3_3

3.2 Best Practices to Manage Skilled Human Resources

For any organization or laboratory to survive in the current competitive scenario, the business strategy has to be aligned with the organization's human resource practices so as to achieve the strategic goals of the organization. Also, since this is an era of technological advancement, hence, it is essential to keep pace with the changing environment and to further develop best practices to increase the efficiency of work at reduced costs.

New technologies and rearrangement of the skills in tune with these technologies is a fundamental requirement. Proactive human resources management along with cultivation of civic and spiritual values for their sustenance and developing disciplined work habits is essential to achieve the above-mentioned change in order to meet the challenges of today and the future [1].

3.2.1 Proactive Habits That Can Increase Productivity of the Youth While Working in the Laboratory

Productivity is very important for any kind of work, especially while working in a laboratory. There are a number of tasks that need to be performed throughout the day, which consume most of the productive hours of the day, ultimately leading to reduced productivity in the laboratory. Taking this into consideration, there are some guidelines, which can be followed keeping in mind the day-to-day routine and this can be used for long-term productivity goals. The guidelines have been summarized in 10 points (Fig. 3.1).

3.2.1.1 Planning the Day in Advance

Preparation of a to-do list the day before which will help in visualizing the upcoming day. Overviewing the tasks listed and ticking them once they are accomplished, gives a sense of accomplishment for a productive day. Penning down the task list streamlines the mental functioning and objectives and promotes creative tasks. A well-planned day further leads to a well-planned week and month, and thus helps in achievement of goals as per the timeline.

3.2.1.2 Time Tracking

A lot of time spent on each task should be prepared as this helps in understanding where and how time is being utilized during the day. When a specific time is allotted to each task, it helps in better scheduling. Therefore, if doing a task is taking longer, it is an indication that there is a mistake in the process. For doing important yet boring tasks like cleaning the instruments, a specific time of the day to do those tasks should be set.

3.2.1.3 Utilization of Spare Time

While doing experiments, there is time in between, often defined as the incubation time, which can be utilized in tasks like data entry, analysis of data, admin work,

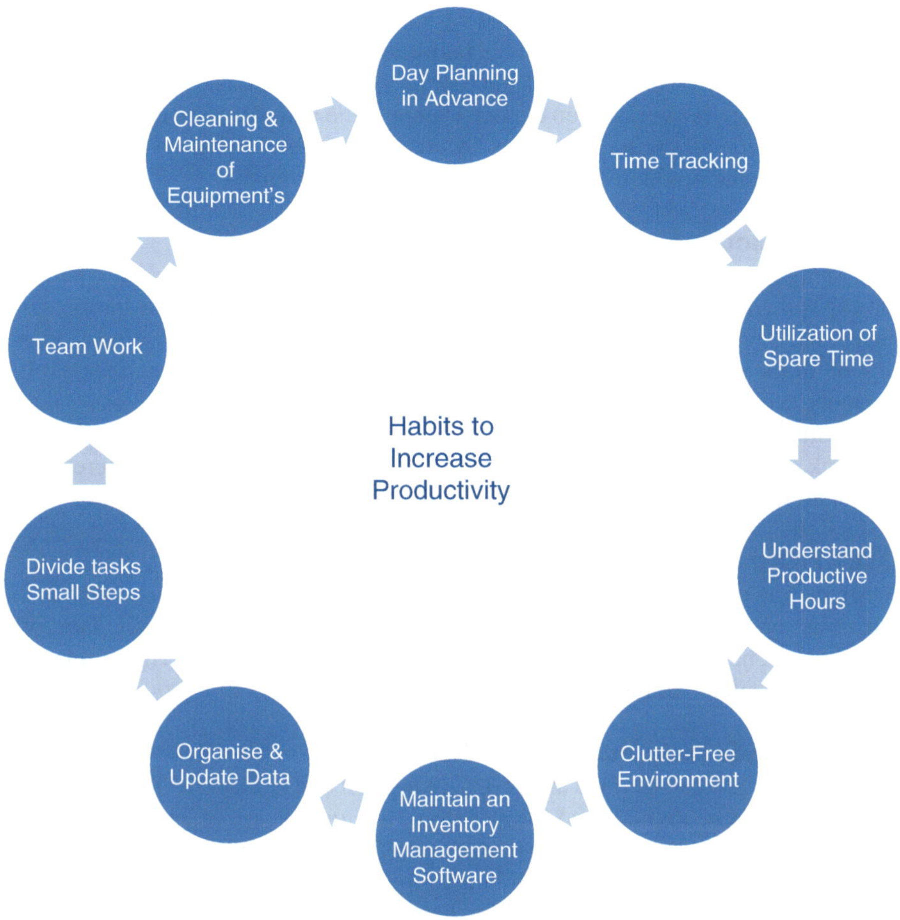
Day Planning in Advance
Time Tracking
Utilization of Spare Time
Understand Productive Hours
Clutter-Free Environment
Maintain an Inventory Management Software
Organise & Update Data
Divide tasks Small Steps
Team Work
Cleaning & Maintenance of Equipment's
Habits to Increase Productivity

Fig 3.1 Human habits to increase productivity in lab

and to prepare buffers needed later in the experiment. It will prevent the loss of valuable time.

3.2.1.4 Understand Productive Hours

An individual has to evaluate a defined time during the day which is more productive for him/her. If the individual is a "morning person" then he/she should reach the laboratory early for work, and if the individual works better later in the day, then he/she should schedule lighter tasks for the morning hours and should leave the tasks that need more concentration for afternoon and evening. Knowing each individual's capacity will not only increase the individual productivity, but will also increase the productivity of the laboratory.

3.2.1.5 Clutter-Free Environment

A workstation that is cluttered with half-empty beakers, pipettes, tissue paper, MCTs, papers, etc. will give very little room for actual work. Therefore, it is recommended to keep the workstation clean by keeping the material back after use, cleaning the beakers, arranging the papers by creating a proper filing system. This will help increase the productivity and creativity of the individual.

3.2.1.6 Maintain an Inventory Management Software

Not being able to find the material or losing it when an individual wants to perform an experiment hampers productivity in the lab. Therefore, it is crucial for the managers, the QA or the administrative staff to create a system of labelling and accounting of all the materials available in the laboratory with their batch number, expiry, quantity, etc. which would help the study personnel to identify the necessary material easily and to notify in advance if a certain material is about to get over or is out of stock. Once the tracking of the material is systematic, it would help increase the productivity of the personnel, and thus maintain GLP standards.

3.2.1.7 Organize and Update Data

Once the material is organized, keeping the data and daily records organized is the next big step toward increasing productivity. Once the experiment is over, data entry should be done as soon as possible. The data should be kept in the right folder and should be available to the right people when needed.

3.2.1.8 Divide Tasks into Smaller Steps

Dividing the task can be done at 2 levels, individual and managerial levels. An individual task can be divided into smaller steps, like in the case of an experiment. At the managerial level, the idea is to divide the task based on the skills and time available with the individuals. This can boost productivity and teamwork, both in one shot. Everyone should be encouraged to help one another and everyone in the laboratory should be sufficiently trained. This would increase productivity in the laboratory as every individual would do the task best suited to their skills.

3.2.1.9 Teamwork

Helping and working together in the laboratory, offering help to others, and giving tips when required, raises the morale and productivity of an individual and the group in the laboratory. A competitive environment in the laboratory should be avoided. Instead, the mindset of working together toward the same goal or a similar outcome will make the individuals support each other.

3.2.1.10 Cleaning and Maintenance of Equipment

Another task that is avoided in the laboratory after finishing the experiment is cleaning the equipment, the bench or keeping the instruments back at their respective places. This has to be done after conducting the experiment or at least before the day ends. This would help keep the laboratory clean, help other team members use it with ease and prepare and set things out for the following day. Adhering to these ten simple steps will help increase the productivity of an individual and a laboratory in the short term, and in turn help an individual be more effective in the long run. It is essential to take these steps and use them effectively in the lab. If one masters these tips, it will not only make them more productive, but also more GLP oriented.

Apart from adoption of good habits, development of communication skills to minimize the gap of understanding, training, and skill development for the adoption of best practices, exposure to additional laboratories working in the same area, use of advanced technology, behavioral changes, work ethics, and practice of yoga plays an important role for an individual to manage his/her work. It also improves the work culture and overall productivity of the laboratory.

3.3 Communication Among the Team Members for Youth-Oriented GLP (YOG)

The most basic aspect of research is the way researchers communicate as it can affect the outcome of the research work. When there is a failure in team communication, it degrades the team's performance and increases errors significantly [2]. Therefore, it is an essential requirement to have a good channel of communication between all the team members including the study director, Principal Investigator (PI), quality assurance staff, the researchers, the technical staff, the administrative staff, and the study personnel, so that all the findings are reported and all the stages of the study are appropriately observed. All the means of communication should be effective and documented before the start of the study, and each person involved in the study needs to be aware of their roles and responsibilities. This is even more important in case of multi-site studies. Inevitably, all variations from the study should be swiftly communicated and any issue confronted in laboratory should be well documented [3].

Management at multiple levels between the study personnel and quality assurance staff is important to have a transparent and frank communication and authority, so that the Principal Investigator and the other management team can carry out GLP and their responsibilities effectively. A written document should be maintained for this.

In multi-center and multi-site studies, a defined authority and communication should be maintained between the team PI, QA, study director, other staff, and study personnel so that everyone has a clear understanding of each activity involved.

In the studies where the responsibilities are delegated to the PI(s), the study director will depend on the individuals to ensure that the relevant phase/s of the study are conducted in line with the study design, relevant standard operating process, and GLP principles. The PI should communicate to the study director about any incident that affects the purpose of the study design defined. A written document should be maintained for this as well.

At every stage of the study, communication is essential between the team PI, study director, and QA. Communication possibly involves:

- Effective participation with QA, i.e., study design including the new SOPs and the revised SOPs should be regularly reviewed, meetings should be attended by the QA team so that problems related to GLP can be resolved.

- The QA personnel should respond to survey and audit reports on time, so that remedial actions are suitably provided in response to inspection/audit findings.

An effective communication channel and a clear line of work allocation can help avoid many problems which can occur in multi-site studies among the study director, sponsor, principal investigator(s), management staff, quality assurance staff, and study personnel at their respective locations.

The study director should also inform all the stakeholders about the progress of the study at all the sites. The study director should also maintain an appropriate communication system between each PI and themselves. For example, it would be advisable to verify the mobile number, landline number, Email ID of all the people involved in the study. It is also advisable to check the mobile signal strength at rural stations, taking into account the difference in time zone and have a language interpreter if needed.

Necessary findings about the QA of the test site should be communicated by the student to the PI of the study and other team members. A written documentation of all the communication and findings should be maintained for future reference.

3.3.1 Advantages of Good Communication Between Team Members

- Good communication plays a vital role in ensuring better productivity at the workplace and improves the relationships among team members. Effective communication reduces the gaps in understanding and also results in better coordination among the team members.
- Showing empathy and open-mindedness while listening attentively at the same time, results in good relationships with the team members.
- Nurturing effective communications skills fosters trust among the members, resolves conflicts, provides better clarity. It boosts satisfaction among the members so that they are better engaged in the jobs handled by them. A team built on these qualities has better productivity.
- Good communication between the team helps the team members share their knowledge effectively with each other (Fig. 3.2).

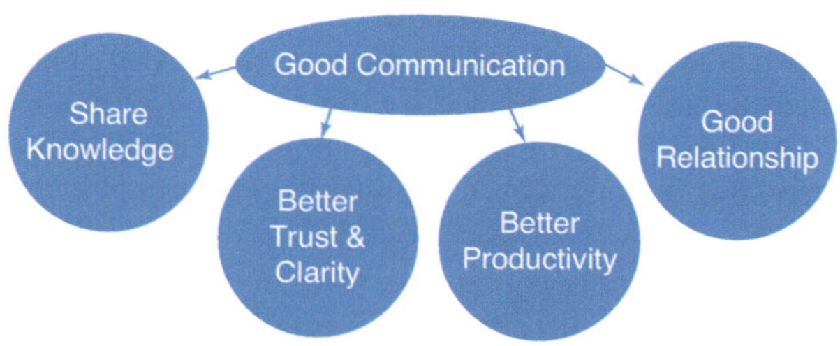

Fig. 3.2 Advantages of good communication

The aspects that improve communication are attentive listening skills, documentation (SOPs, DRSs, etc.), open conversation among the team members, and honest feedback on the discussions/issues among the team members. Use of technology can also aid communication.

3.4 Organizational Structure and Its Importance in GLP

An organization chart is required in GLP to understand the overall structure of the test facility. This gives an idea of how the facility is functioning. The organizational structure chart comes under the quality manual for any organization as it is an important document. These documents can also incorporate the following details related to each individual:

- Biodata
- Records of the training attended
- Detailed description of the job role

All the 3 documents together are required to maintain individual records for GLP. It is important as it demonstrates that the staff working have the ability, qualification, experience, and necessary training to execute the task at hand. To align these documents to GLP, the content and format of these records should be documented and specified in SOPs and should be validated by QA audits regularly [4–6]. Example in Fig. 3.3.

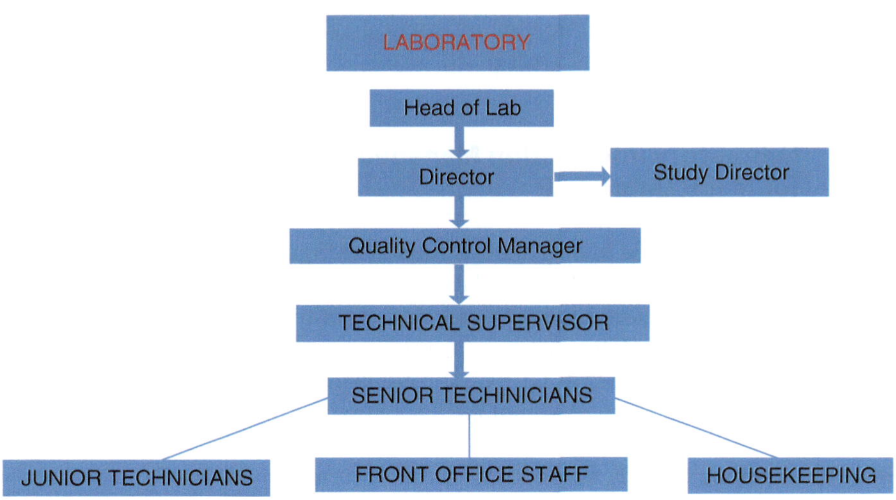

Fig. 3.3 Example of the laboratory Organizational Structure

3.5 Quality Management System and Its Importance in Development of Skilled Human Resource

The potential advantages of implementing a quality control framework based on International Standards for a laboratory and research organization are the ability to reliably deliver publications, products, and services that satisfy Institute's expectations and relevant legislative and regulatory requirements. This, in turn, is also important for the development of skilled human resources and career advancement.

3.6 Role of Technology in Skill Development Youth-Oriented GLP (YOG)

Good Laboratory Practices involve the analysis, development, and management of quality, which includes the expansion of Standard Operating Procedures (SOPs), specimen, study, documents, and release methods for the laboratory work. According to Good Laboratory Practice, testing is monitored by an independent quality assurance staff in the laboratory. The process is expensive but it should be incorporated in laboratories and research organizations. The comprehensive responsibility of the regime with GLP principles remains with the appointed skilled in charge. Individuals should have a traceable written procedure for all the chemicals, materials, and reagents necessary for the work to proceed smoothly. Responsibility of a QA should be performed by a person who is not a part of the specific responsibility for that particular function, who is not a member of the investigating team.

Worldwide the role of technology in complying with Good Laboratory Practices is increasing. Information technology (IT) helps to gather and store the data and also helps maintain the quality and safety of data [7]. Information technology (IT) has revolutionized the way data is transferred by decreasing the time it takes to generate the test results and creating an opportunity to work on large datasets in research work with minimum errors [3, 8].

3.6.1 Laboratory Information Management System for Maintaining GLP

A Laboratory Information Management System (LIMS) is a software that allows one to successfully manage samples and data to enhance laboratory efficiency. It also helps in tracking data associated with samples, experiments, laboratory workflows, and instruments [3, 9]. LIMS software supports the laboratories in complying with the regulatory specifications such as GLP by encapsulating how and what has been done, thus enabling efficient management of the laboratory. LIMS helps in the following:

- **Data Tracking and Trending**: LIMS stores information of tested samples, their outcome, and all the related records of the participants.

- **SOPs and DRSs**: LIMS helps in the creation of SOPs and DRSs and in maintaining its records.
- **Employee and Student Data:** With LIMS, all the data for employees and students can be managed in one place and this information is available at a click. It works as a tracking tool for those who need training and can be done remotely as well.
- **Synthesis:** The study result can be captured directly from the equipment used, and the same can be fed into the computer system, minimizing error, and enhancing accuracy.
- **Master Record Keeping:** LIMS is an essential tool to maintain and generate accurate reports on time. Reports can be automated so that the system can generate reports regularly on a daily, weekly, and monthly basis.
- **Labelling:** Helps in generating automatic labels in a similar format for all the samples and inventory of the laboratory.
- **Inventory Management:** Keeping records of the inventory is one of the main functions in the management of any laboratory. LIMS system has fully automated the process of inventory management, while ensuring that chemicals, equipment, kits, etc. are ordered in advance as per the requirement. It prevents any delays in the laboratory workflow.
- **Quality Control:** Centralized access and storage of quality control data help in providing the highest level of quality.

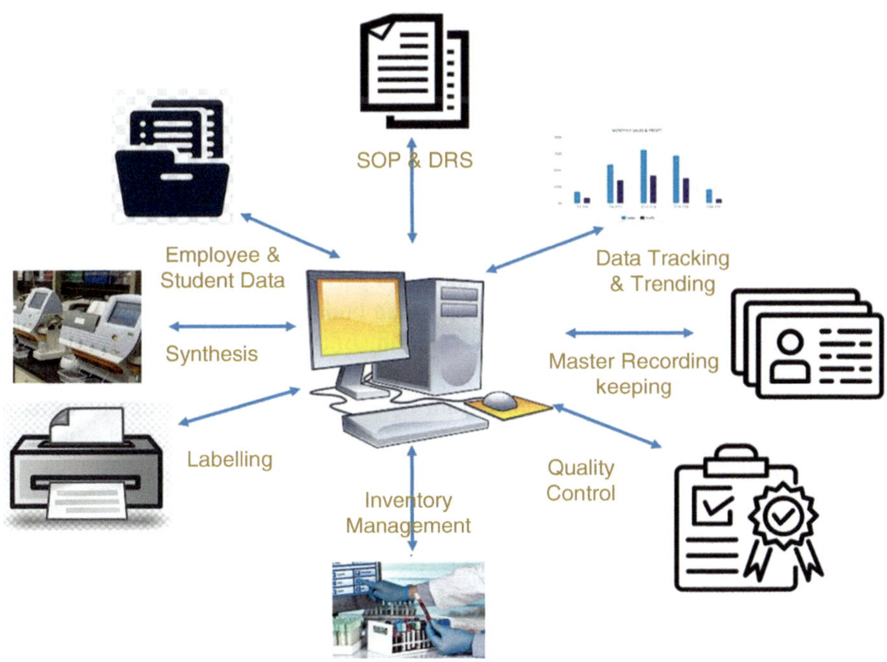

Fig. 3.4 Benefits of a Laboratory Information Management System

Laboratory Information Management System supports in three main ways:

- Perfection—LIMS helps the laboratories produce perfect and repeatable results.
- Effectiveness—LIMS supports the laboratories to automatize, speed up, and make the difficult job easy.
- Management—LIMS helps the laboratories accumulate and recover the outcome very quickly (Fig. 3.4).

3.7 Importance of Training and Team Building Workshops in GLP

Training in a laboratory is important as it is aimed at improving the proficiency of an individual as it provides him the knowledge on how to execute the procedures necessary to do the prescribed task. It can be significant from indicative understanding, which is understanding of reality or undeviating information. Generally, the goal of a training program in the laboratory defines the success of a training program, which are:

- Transfer to the work situation (generality).
- Long-term use of what was learned for the job (maintenance).
- Structured training programs are made for trainees to learn individually or in a team.
- Focused training is given to individuals or groups for a particular position and role.
- Training is given to teams who are then returned to their job situations (where the trainees work alone or as a part of a team, which may be nested in a network of teams).
- Training may be delivered to a group at a particular site, and then they can be returned to their own job site.
- Training of teams can be defined as training in which teams are used to increase procedural knowledge and skills of individuals to do a specific job.
- For comprehensive team achievement, individual methodology, knowledge, and proficiency are important in functioning as a part of teamwork.
- Training the team is a different process than building a team, which happens at the actual job location and focuses on scrutiny of the teamwork, its activities, and procedures to improve the productivity of the team as a whole.
- Training the team is also different from cooperative learning, as this happens in schools and colleges and its prime focus is on explanatory knowledge rather than the knowledge of methodology and procedures which helps in attaining proficiency.

3.8 Imbibing Work Ethical Behavior in Youth

Ignorance and lack of discourse lead to unethical practices. Ethical conduct is important to preserve the integrity of the research work done by the individual and institutes. It is important to imbibe ethical behavior among youth as per GLP standards for advancement in research [10]. There are certain ethical principles that should be followed for imbibing work ethic behavior in youth:

- Honesty—In scientific communications, honesty is always important. Fabricated, false, or misrepresented data should not be presented. Data and results should be presented honestly with proper result, method, process, and procedure. Fraud should not be done with sponsors, researchers, co-workers or public in general.
- Objectivity—Attempt to avoid any bias in experimental design, data interpretation, data analysis, review, etc.
- Integrity—Strive to keep agreements and promises, and one should act with sincerity.
- Carefulness—One should critically and carefully examine the work done and avoid any kind of careless errors and negligence in the research work like data records and data collection.
- Openness—One should be open to new ideas and criticism.
- Intellectual Property—One should honor other person's rights, patents, licence, copyrights, or any other form of intellectual property. Due recognition should be given to all the contributors in the study. Unpublished data, methodology, and results should not be used without permission.
- Confidentiality—Confidentiality in communications should be maintained such as during submission of grants or manuscripts.
- Responsible Publication—Published data should be such that it helps in advancement of the research and benefits to everyone and not just the individual.
- Responsible Mentoring—The mentors should advise, educate, and mentor students in such a manner that they are able to make their own decisions.
- Social Responsibility—Attempt to promote social advancement of the society and prevent any harm through research to the society.
- Non-Discrimination—Avoid any kind of discrimination against the students or fellow workers on the basis of sex, religion, etc.
- Legality—Institutes and governmental laws and policies should be obeyed.
- Animal Care—Animals used for the research work should be given proper care and respect and should not be sacrificed without any objective.
- Protection of human subjects—When humans are taken in research as participants the researchers should respect their dignity and privacy. Minimize any risks or harm to the human subjects.

3.9 Zero Effect-Zero Defect Youth Oriented GLP (ZED-YOG)

Management programs such as ZED have been implemented by the Government of India. ZED has a culture with a bi-focus approach toward the customers on one side and the society of the other side. Zero defect means that the quality of the product from a patent is very high and is error free. Zero effect means that there should be no negative effect on the environment due to manufacturing. This highlights the government's ardent desire to pay particular attention to manufacturing as a means to promote sustainable growth in order to transform the course of the economy. ZED can be clubbed with Youth-Oriented GLP (YOG), which will help inspire today's skilled youth to implement quality standards in the laboratories and other research works [11].

Zero Defect, Zero Effect is useful to examine the competitiveness of the youth, a business, a region, and a country as a whole. For the improvement of productivity and environment protection, the roles of young generation taking initiative in business strategies, polices, and knowledge economic development for maximizing productivity needs to recast to fully taped dormant potentials. Productivity is the key to any country's growth. In today's world, incorporating concern for the environment is essential along with expanding productivity, continuous improvement and achievement.

3.10 Importance of Skill Development in GLP

3.10.1 Benefits to the Individual

- Individual requirement—On the job, learning boosts confidence and helps one to perform and handle the task better.
- Increases Reputation—A person with knowledge is an asset to the laboratory and earns more respect and regards in the team.
- Stress free working—Once a person gains knowledge on the task, the work for him becomes easier and enjoyable, which leads to better productivity and stress-free working.

3.10.2 Benefits to the Laboratory

- Laboratory requirements—Every laboratory requires the work force to have a minimum standard of knowledge and skills for an individual to handle specialized tasks.
- Safety—A knowledgeable individual is able to handle an emergency situation more carefully and with greater responsibility.
- Rotation between different job functions—Knowledgeable individuals trained in different skills can easily switch between different tasks at the time of deadlines.
- Minimize attrition rate—When the individuals' knowledge is upgraded on a regular basis, it helps in minimizing the attrition rate as well.

3.11 Suggestions for Training and Skill Upgradation

3.11.1 Suggestions for Individuals

- Individuals should always be on the lookout for new training opportunities in the laboratory. It can include learning a new technique or skill by the institute, Principal Investigator, other team members, workshops, seminars, conferences, or any other such programs.
- Individuals should look out for Internet-based e-learning programs, as they not only save time but also keeps them updated with new technologies and techniques.

- An individual should have reverence toward the instruments, machines, and tools that they use, as it is the source and means to achieve the assigned tasks, and should also develop an urge to know more about them.

3.11.2 Suggestions for the Laboratory

- The laboratory should encourage growth and knowledge development through training and skill upgradation. Skilled individuals are always an asset to a laboratory in the long run.
- Skill development helps in increasing the productivity and in preventing an exodus of trained individuals. Individuals would like to stay in a laboratory, which has good training and skill development policies.
- Training and skill development is a win–win situation for both, the laboratory and the individual. It is beneficial at all stages of an individual's career as there is always a scope of learning more than what you already know.

Learning something new every day should become a part of GLP, which will enhance individual skills regularly.

3.12 Role of Yoga and Meditation to Inculcate Values in the Performance and Dedication to Work

Human resource is the most important asset of a laboratory, as it plays a great role in the performance and productivity of the laboratory. Spiritual enhancement focuses on development of morals or civic sense, principles, character, and innovation of an individual which is important for a multi ethnic and multidisciplinary GLP facility. Spirituality also helps in developing an attitude of integrity and for attainment of a healthy eco system in the lab. Spirituality, as opposed to religion, is an intangible asset that motivates the individual and allows him/her to concentrate better, bring positivity and connectedness at workplace. Thus, it helps him/her to perform his/her best, and attain work satisfaction which results in reduction of the attrition rate. Being an intangible factor, it motivates the work force and eventually creates job satisfaction leading to retention of employees. Spirituality helps an employee or an individual attain certain values to serve the community, society, country, and world as a whole through the organization's setup which helps in long-term correction in the prevailing conditions. Studies show that there is an association between spirituality at the workplace, performance, and job contentment [6, 12].

Adopting spirituality at the work place helps the personnel in vertical and horizontal growth, both. A spiritual path at the workplace helps both the organization and the individual to prosper and advance in academic-social responsibility. Others argue that this is useful in being truthful toward one's own self and develop care and empathy for all the fellow workers and society. It is an attempt to live a valuable life and perform better at work. It is said that spirituality in management is important as it helps run an organization better, more efficiently, and effectively while attaining core contentment, happiness, and success at work at the same time [9].

3.13 Future Directions and Clinical Implications

Doctors, researchers, and other healthcare professionals should be given alternative venues of training like communication skills, laboratory information management system, zero effect–zero defect youth-oriented GLP adopted by Neuroscience Research Lab, PGIMER, Chandigarh, practical procedures and clinical examination. This would help in enhancing patient care in clinical environment. Therefore, in the future, an appropriate planning is required for successful training of healthcare professionals [13, 14].

Acknowledgment Dr. Akshay Anand, Neuroscience Research Laboratory, Department of Neurology, PGIMER, Chandigarh-160012, India.

References

1. Lakhotia SC. Research and innovation in universities – why and how should these be promoted? 2019 August.
2. Sabando RC, Belli S. Communication problems during laboratory work: interaction professor-student and student-student. J Interpers Relat Intergroup Relat Identity. Winter 2017;10:81–93.
3. Okay Somerville B, Scholarios D. A multilevel examination of skills-oriented human resource management and perceived skill utilization during recession implications for the well being of all workers. Hum Resour Manag. 2019 Mar;58(2):139–54.
4. World Health Organization. Good laboratory practice training manual: for the trainee: a tool for training and promoting good laboratory practice (GLP) concepts in disease endemic countries. World Health Organization; 2010 Feb 2.
5. Giovannini E. Human resources management and training: compilation of good practices in statistical offices. New York and Geneva: United Nations; 2013.
6. Hassan M, Bin Nadeem A, Akhter A. Impact of workplace spirituality on job satisfaction: mediating effect of trust. Cogent Bus Manag. 2016;3(1):1189808.
7. Sachdeva G. Impact of spirituality in management: a review. In: Science and spirituality for a sustainable world: emerging research and opportunities. Pennsylvania: IGI Global; 2019. p. 1–22.
8. Stokes T. Good laboratory practice and information technology in the '90s. Chemom Intell Lab Syst. 1993;21(2):131–8.
9. McDowall RD. Chapter 6 Laboratory information management systems. In: Comprehensive analytical chemistry, vol. 39. New York: Elsevier; 2003. p. 287–325.
10. Behal B, Chaddah P, Chandrasekaran S, Gardia A, Ghosh A, Godbole R. Ethics in science education, research and governance. New Delhi: Indian National Science Academy; 2019.
11. Tyagi R, Anand A. Development and implementation of ZED-YOG quality module: Niyantrita Madhumeha Bharata skill development initiatives. Ann Neurosci. 2019;26(1):37–44.
12. Forest JC, Rheault C, Dang-Vu TK. The laboratory information system (LIS): I-application to the clinical chemistry laboratory. Clin Biochem. 1985;18(2):78–84.
13. Dent JA. Current trends and future implications in the developing role of clinical skills centres. Med Teach. 2001 Sep;23(5):483–9.
14. LeRoy L, Kalfoglou AL, Wolman DM, editors. Medicare laboratory payment policy: now and in the future. Washington, DC: National Academies Press; 2001 Jan 4.

Operationalization of Research SOPs for PhD Scholars

4

Priya Mehra, Gillipsie Minhas, and Winston Costa Pereira

4.1 Introduction

Standard Operating Procedures (SOPs) are detailed, written instructions that aim to achieve uniformity while performing work functions [1, 2]. The aim of an SOP is to comply with regulations, maintain standards of quality, and mitigate safety and health risks in a consistent and efficient manner, thus overcoming the risk of variability and achieving trust and satisfaction in the process [3].

Good laboratory practice (GLP) is a quality system implemented to ensure quality, reliability, reproducibility, uniformity, and consistency. The concept of GLP came into existence in 1976 [4], which was prior to the GLP FDA mandated requirements on June 20, 1979, thus ensuring integrity in research [5]. In general, GLP can be defined as a set of principles that define standard operating procedures (SOPs), data recording sheet (DRS), raw data entry, maintenance of records, sample verification, sample record, log sheets, and many other routine activities that may require validation at any stage of research. Studies have indicated that research and training without any standard procedures may result in research malpractices [6] and

Priya Mehra and Gillipsie Minhas contributed equally with all other contributors.

P. Mehra
Department of Biotechnology, Panjab University, Chandigarh, India

Neuroscience Research Lab, Department of Neurology, PGIMER, Chandigarh, Chandigarh, India

G. Minhas
Neuroscience Research Lab, Department of Neurology, PGIMER, Chandigarh, Chandigarh, India

W. Costa Pereira (✉)
Regulatory Submissions Specialists, Toronto, ON, Canada
e-mail: winston@regulatorysubmissions.ca

A. Anand (ed.), *Quality Assurance Implementation in Research Labs*,
https://doi.org/10.1007/978-981-16-3074-3_4

conflicts, while other studies have also highlighted the importance of GLP in a research laboratory [7].

SOPs are considered as the building blocks of the GLP system. They ensure that the study is conducted, documented, and recorded for compliance. Data has shown that non-usage of SOPs may invariably lead to failure of experimental protocols, erroneous processes, higher variability than expected, and lack of proper oversight [8]. It was shown that in the early 1970s, FDA investigated several cases pertaining to poor practice in toxicology laboratories throughout the USA. Therefore, in this chapter, we highlight the use and implementation of SOPs to produce reliable and reproducible results, and as a valuable training tool for doctoral students, not just to toxicity testing for which these are originally designed.

4.2 SOP and Its Attributes in the Quality Management System

The main attributes in a Quality Management System (QMS) include Quality Assurance (QA) and documentation for a wide array of institutions such as biotechnology, academic, pharmaceutical, hospitals, diagnostic setups, and clinical laboratories. Both Quality Control (QC) and Quality Assurance (QA) form a part of the Quality Management System. QA has a wider scope in the process, and is mainly involved in providing confidence to all the stakeholders concerned that the product (or patent) will perform as expected [9, 10]. As mentioned, Quality Assurance is known to be a proactive process and is active in preventing flaws in the process. However, Quality Control (QC) focuses on identifying a defect.

The chief component of Quality Assurance in research laboratories is a process that involves written instructions that describe the operations which need to be performed. This document is known as the Standard Operating Procedures (SOP). In a clinical and pharmaceutical operation, the quality assurance units are responsible for surveying the operations in accordance with the SOP, and for ensuring that the generated data satisfies the requirements for quality [11, 12]. As far as clinical trials are concerned, SOPs are represented by the study protocols used in the trial. GCP (Good Clinical Practice) is further characterized by ethical principles, which is primarily aimed at protecting the personal integrity and welfare of the trial subjects. The Declaration of Helsinki is the accepted basis for clinical trial ethics for planning, conducting, surveying, and evaluating clinical trials, which is the cornerstone of GCP.

4.3 Lifecycle of an SOP

The lifecycle of an SOP includes an SOP of SOPs that describes how the life cycle of any SOP is managed from its inception to retirement. It provides the readers with an explanation of how the SOPs are used.

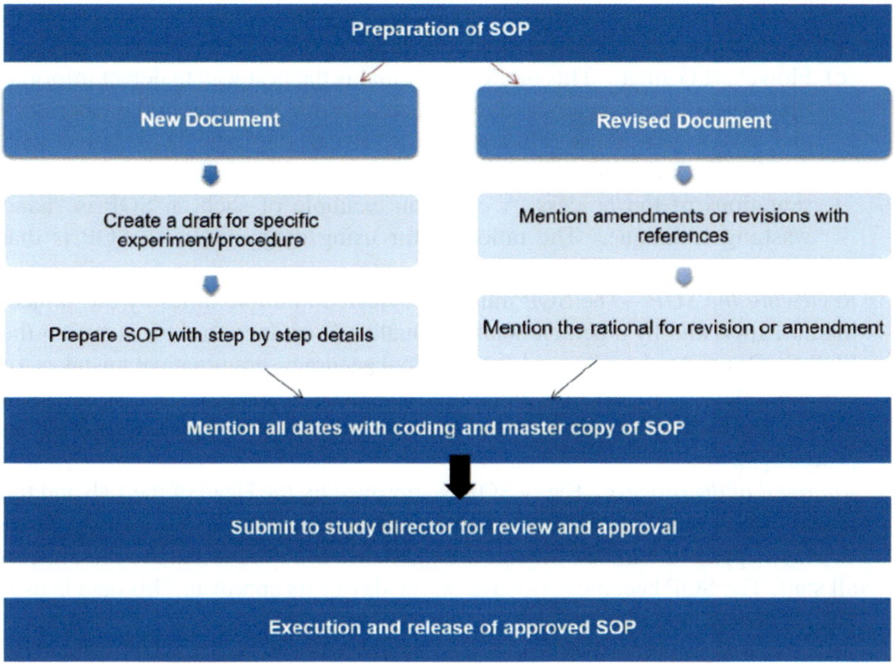

Fig. 4.1 Summary of life cycle of an SOP

For any amendments in the SOP, the user must mention all the details with a justification of why it is required, its importance, and the possible outcome. The revised SOP should contain all the details with their rationale and justification. This should be done and reviewed by the management system [9]. The life cycle of an SOP occurs in the following six stages (Fig. 4.1):

1. *Initiation of a new SOP*—Whenever a new SOP is required, a request is sent to the Departmental Head. In a research laboratory, this may be required when a new procedure is to be implemented, when new equipment is installed and people are to be trained properly by the vendor, or when there is a particular requirement by the regulatory agencies, due to the initiation of guidelines and regulations. There must be a form with the Quality Assurance that implicates the requirement/change in the SOP. The person who requests it (or an RTI activist) must give suitable justification for the purpose and rationale for creating the SOP. This will aid the approval process. The Head will then have a meeting with all the stakeholders and the Quality Head before signing the approval process.
2. *Drafting a new SOP*—Possible ways of drafting an SOP are as follows:
   (a) Simple Steps Format—These are short procedures that do not involve multiple subheadings. It can be written as short bullet points or a numbered section.
   (b) Hierarchical Steps Format—Around 90% of institutions around the world follow this process. This process is suitable for lengthy procedures where

multiple steps are required. This process may have sections and subsections that are numbered in chronological order.

   (c) Flowchart Format—This particular format is the best way to depict information as it is easily understandable. Such a format is placed in the laboratory and serves as a quick reference guide. Every step may be depicted with block arrows that are a part of a written chart or have diagrammatic representations of the process. A common example of such an SOP is "hand washing technique." The rationale for using diagrams in an SOP is that visual aids can be followed easily.

3. *Reviewing the SOP*—The SOP must be reviewed multiple times by the subject matter expert and by a person (such as Quality Assurance) tasked to review the SOP. SOPs need to be reviewed for technical accuracy, grammatical mistakes, or any other flaws that affect the authenticity of the process. An SOP has to reflect the process as it is done and should not be a hypothetical representation of the process [7].
4. *Approval of the process*—Every SOP is approved by the Head of the Lab and the Quality Head. The approved SOP is then sent to the Quality Management Team to get an approval number. This gets logged into the system that is accessible to all staff. The SOP becomes effective on the day of its approval. This date is usually on the last page of the SOP.
5. *Revision and Revision History*—An SOP has a lifespan of 2 years. When the SOP needs to be revised, a request is sent to the Lab Head either from the subject matter expert (in cases of revision before the due date), or from the Quality Management (QM) team. This request is in the form of a Change Request or any other procedure followed within the organization. Any amendments to the SOP must detail the rationale for it. In clinical trials, GCP guidelines must be implemented to ensure the quality of the study. The GCPs constitute a standard system for planning, conducting, and monitoring the clinical study in compliance with GCP guidelines and applicable regulations [10].
6. *Decommissioning, where the SOP is no longer required and is retired from use*—Obsolete SOPs are to be removed from circulation and decommissioned. All decommissioned SOPs are stored in the archive section under the control of the Documentation Control personnel. This person can be under the direct control of the QA, or it can be a separate department. The archived SOPs are kept for a period of 2 years or more, as per the requirements of the regulations.

4.4 Regulatory Requirements

In the pharmaceutical industry, it is mandatory to follow guidelines and implement a QMS that includes SOPs. In research laboratories, this can be voluntary. In the mid-1970s, the US FDA first implemented GLP guidelines to define the minimum standards to conduct nonclinical studies to generate high-quality and reliable data [13]. The final GLP regulations were later published on December 22, 1978, which became law on June 20, 1979 [14]. Later in 1981, GLP principles were adopted by the Organization for Economic Co-operation and Development (OECD), an intergovernmental organization formed to avoid different systems of implementation that could hinder international trade [15]. In 1997, the US FDA published International Conference on Harmonization guidelines (ICH) on clinical studies in the federal register (Vol 62, No. 90). The FDA documented many flaws in clinical and nonclinical research, such as poorly trained study directors or personnel who are executing the protocol. Some studies have shown that poor study design/malpractices or generation of improper raw data leads to the misconduct of research and failure to establish quality. These failures may include a lack of standardization of specific protocols, inadequate resources, and instruments that lack periodic calibration and maintenance. Therefore, the FDA requires that research is done under compliance and be back-traceable wherever required [16–19].

The ICH guidelines for quality are approved by the European Medicines Evaluation Agency (EMEA), USFDA, and the Japanese Ministry of Health (MHW). These guidelines include the requirements for SOPs. Furthermore, the 21CFR58 (Code of Federal Regulations, Title 21--Food and Drugs; Part 58--Good Laboratory Practice for Nonclinical Laboratory Studies) describes the SOP preparation and implementation of different routine procedures [20]. On the other hand, the US Environmental Protection Agency (EPA) provides detailed guidance for developing SOPs (EPA QA/G-6; EPA/600/B-07/001). As per these guidelines, SOPs describe both technical and fundamental operational elements of an organization that would be managed under a work plan or a QA Project Plan [EPA Requirements for QA Project Plans (QA/R-5) (EPA 2001a)], or Chap. 5 of the EPA Quality Manual for Environmental Programs, (EPA Manual 5360 A) and under an organization's Quality Management Plan [EPA Requirements for Quality Management Plans (QA/R-2) (EPA 2001b)], or Chap. 3 of the EPA Quality Manual [21]. The ISO 9000 standards are not considered a regulation or guideline issued by the government; however, different industries have followed this generic quality management framework. Different sections of ISO 9000 guidelines have been known to emphasize the need for written procedures or SOPs [22]. As per the ISO 9001:2015 guidelines, an SOP is a policy and procedure document that describes the regular and recurring activities appropriate to quality operations [23]. Established SOPs add value to the organizations for maintaining a quality system and documentation. The ISO 9001:2015 SOP guidelines define the specific formats for designing, documentation, template, and presentation. This helps an organization to establish control systems and quality management [24].

4.5 Regulations of the SOP

4.5.1 FDA Guidelines

Form 483 is issued to a responsible person in the organization and it comprises a list of objections that are found by the FDA auditor as part of the compliance issues. The US FDA has noted that the main cause of observations found in Form 483 observations and Warning Letters is due to an inadequately crafted SOP. This Form can also be called as a prerequisite to a Warning Letter. A Warning Letter is the final warning to a company that has significantly violated its regulatory policies. Corrective actions must be taken on part of the company management to comply with the FDA regulations. Specific SOP issues can be traced back to poor communication. However, it has been recognized that poorly written SOPs can quietly grow into a host of major compliance problems.

FDA has recognized under section 211.100 (**21 CFR, Section 211.100**) [25] that a well-crafted SOP is an absolute necessity in creating a compliant product. SOPs form the basis of every regulatory compliant activity, which in turn forms the backbone of regulatory compliance activities in all companies regulated by Good Manufacturing Practice (GMP) rules and regulations.

4.5.2 Health Canada

Health Canada has introduced Good Manufacturing Practice guidelines, which is part of the Food and Drug Regulations (Part C Division 2). As per Health Canada's Natural Health Product Regulation (NHPR) Sections 49 and 50 (**Natural Health Product Regulations, Health Canada**) [26, 27], a major deficiency seen in the Operations is the deviation of the Standard Operating Procedure (SOP). Any evidence of GMP compliance is seen in the implementation of a relevant SOP.

Health Canada has mandated several SOPs such as the Good Manufacturing Practices guide for drug products (GUI-0001), which is intended to facilitate GMP compliance by the regulated party with the Food and Drug Act, the regulations, and the applicable administrative policies.

The United States Environmental Protection Agency has also prepared a document called "guidance for preparing SOPs" [28]. This document explains the various steps in writing an SOP.

Checklist for SOP

Checklist serves two purposes, one is to ensure that the steps are followed in correct order and the other is documentation of completed actions. Checklist should be attached to the points in SOP where they are used. There can also be SOPs for preparing checklists.

Quality Management

The Quality Management plan of an organization should have a system of numbering and systematic identification of the SOPs. The SOPs should have a title, revision number, date, and page number. This can help in traceability and maintenance of SOPs.

4.6 Necessity for a New SOP and the Attributes to Create One

Why is it necessary to create a new SOP? The answer lies in the problem and the necessity to create a new protocol to standardize the process. Moreover, the need for SOPs is described in the guidelines discussed previously in this chapter. However, the basic requirement for an SOP arises from the need for a uniform procedure to be used by the end users to establish a standardized protocol [22].

4.7 Types and Content Requirements for a Good SOP

An SOP can be prepared to define a technical or an administrative process followed in an organization. Furthermore, an SOP of SOPs defines the protocol followed in designing and preparing a new SOP. It also includes the guidelines for revision, approval, archival, and distribution of an SOP in various sections [29].

Every SOP is written and designed as per the protocol that might be in house and has passed internal validation, or has been designed by external agencies such as the manufacturers of kits and equipment.

Every new SOP has the following attributes to follow based on the SOP criteria:

1. All SOPs shall be written in Times Roman Font size 12, heading and subheading should be written in boldface. The maximum font size can be14.
2. The sections are numbered with a high level numbering and the subsections are numbered in the lower subsequent order as shown in Fig. 4.2.
   1.0 Heading

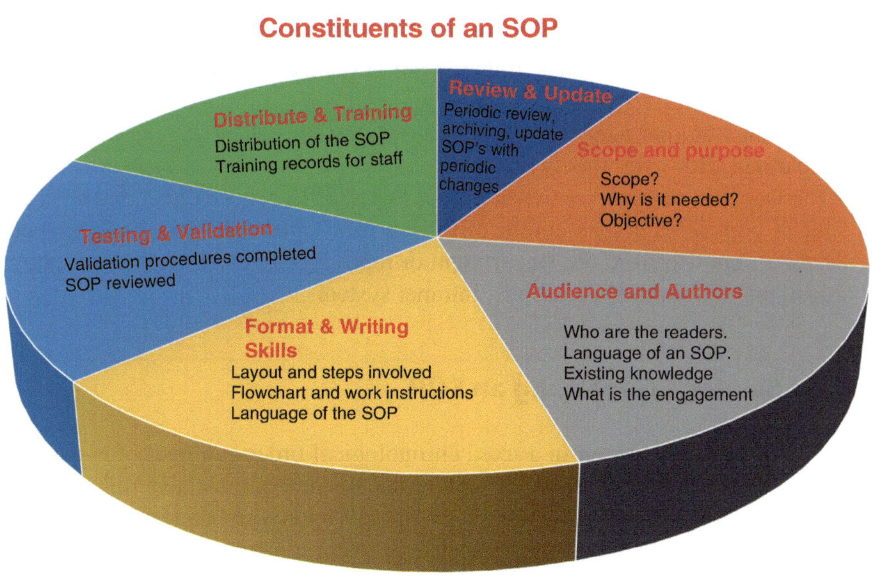

Fig. 4.2 Constituents of an SOP

1.1 Subheading 1
 1.1.1 Subheading 2
  1.1.1.1 Subheading 3
   a. Point 1
   b. Point 2

It must be noted that the first number of every subsequent heading coincides with the last number of the previous section. The distance between the first number and the heading/subheading section must be 0.5 inches.

3. The responsibility section of the SOP shall specify the person and the department responsible for following the SOP and completing all the activities as specified in the SOP.
4. Each SOP should have an effective date and the next revision date.
5. The effective date is the date when the SOP has been finalized and approved by the Lab Head.
6. The training of the staff shall be completed within 10 days from the effective date of the SOP. There must be a Record of Training (ROT) that must be signed by all the staff members who will be following this SOP. The ROT is kept with the Human Resources Department and a copy is kept with the Department. All new employees must be trained according to the SOP prior to active participation in the protocol. The ROT must be signed as a proof of training.
7. All the forms associated with an SOP are a part of the annexure section of the SOP.
8. Each form must have a unique control number. This is administered by the QA and is called a Record Control number. Accountability of every form is important, as it aids in the traceability of forms in case of an investigation or conflict.
9. Every SOP has a unique number called the SOP number. This number is an alphanumeric number consisting of the department name followed by 4–5 numbers, such as SOP-Lab-QC-00001.
10. Every page of the SOP has 2 identification points—the page numbers and the name of the SOP. This avoids confusion.
11. Some institutions may use a crimping mechanism where the pages cannot be separated. However, this is optional.
12. The Department receives two copies of this SOP, they are called controlled copies. A controlled copy stamp is affixed in front of each SOP. This SOP should not be removed from the Department or reproduced in any way. A soft copy is available within the institution's intranet system.

4.8 Sections Governing an SOP

Every SOP must be written in a fixed chronological order and needs to follow the guidelines or recommendations [21]. Every establishment must also follow its own protocol for an SOP and this is termed as an SOP for writing and implementing an SOP (or SOP of SOPs) (Fig. 4.3). However, the consensus and style of writing an SOP, as stated by Isaman V, 1995 should be maintained [30]. A recently published article also defines the development of an SOP and its essential components [31].

a

<table>
<tr><td>Institutional stamp</td><td colspan="3">ABCD
<u>Controlled Document, Not to be Reproduced</u></td></tr>
<tr><td>Departmental Policy</td><td colspan="2">Department: XYZ</td><td>Policy No: 0000000
Version No: 00</td></tr>
<tr><td colspan="3">Title:</td><td>JCI Code:</td></tr>
<tr><td colspan="2">Supersedes: (0000000;
Version 00; Date/Month/Year)</td><td>Copy No:</td><td>Page no.-</td></tr>
</table>

1. **INTRODUCTION**

1.1 All Laboratory staff such as MLA's, MLSO's as well as SMLSO's have to be trained before carrying out activities in the laboratory such as collection, processing, storage and infusion of Hematopoietic Stem Cells.

1.2 Training is given to all concerned Laboratory Staff within the Stem Cell Laboratory (Internal Training) or at an external Location (External Training) in order to maintain the quality and minimize losses of the Stem Cells unit being processed in the Stem Cell Laboratory.

2. **PURPOSE**

2.1 This SOP is designed to address training of all the activities related to Cord Blood Banking as well as Peripheral Blood Stem Cells processing and transplantation.

2.2 Cord Blood Banking is based on a strict acceptance criteria based on established literature, this training is designed to enable the technologist to increase the efficiency of the process.

2.3 The purpose of this SOP is to train new and existing staff members in any new process change or development and to continuously monitor the progress via competency assessment or evaluation.

2.4 To train and update the personnel for better implementation of the SOP's related to laboratory activities, update technical knowledge through lectures in the area that will enhance the theoretical advancement in the field.

2.5 To identify areas of concern that requires training for the better implementation of the SOP.

2.6 It is very strongly encouraged to address any doubts with the Seniors so that proper timely action is taken.

3. **APPLICABILITY**

3.1 This SOP is applicable to working of the Stem Cell Laboratory and must be followed by each staff working on Stem Cell processing and Cryopreservation.

3.2 This SOP is in vogue after the approval and authorization at various levels before its final implementation.

4. **RESPONSIBILITIES**

4.1 All Technical staff (MLA, MLSO, SMLSO)is responsible to follow this process.

4.2 Principal Clinical Scientist is responsible to review and supervise the process.

4.3 The Head of the Blood Bank Division and the Director of the CML are responsible to approve the SOP.

4.4 The CQI Department is responsible to review the SOP and create a Document Control number for the SOP.

4.5 The PSMMC Director is responsible to authorize this SOP.

5. **POLICY**

5.1 This SOP is developed by the Stem Cell Section of PSMMC for the requirement in undertaking safe and effective procedures of storage and transplantation of Peripheral Blood Stem Cells from suitable donors/patients.

5.2 This SOP is compiled by Senior MLSO and Principal Scientist who is in charge of the entire Laboratory Operations.

5.3 This SOP is further reviewed by the Head of the Division and the Director of CML and Blood Bank before it is finally approved by the PSMMC Director.

5.4 This SOP should comply with Good Documentation Practice methods and by International Accreditation Bodies such as Foundation for Accreditation of Cellular Therapy (FACT) and Joint Accreditation Committee for ISCT and EBMT (JACIE).

5.5 This SOP is implemented only after approval and being postal on the Intranet site. A controlled copy is in the Stem Cell section and all previous versions are maintained in the archive.

5.6 The status of SOP's before its final approval will be labelled as 'Draft' version.

5.7 Duplication, Modification to this SOP without proper authorization is prohibited.

Fig. 4.3 (**a**, **b**) Sample SOP

b

Institutional stamp	ABCD Controlled Document, Not to be Reproduced		
Departmental Policy	**Department: XYZ**		**Policy No: 0000000** **Version No: 00**
Title:			**JCI Code:**
Supersedes: (0000000; Version 00; Date/Month/Year)		**Copy No:**	**Page no.-**

5.8 This SOP is compiled as per the Hospital wide policy for the management of Policy and Procedures.

6. **PROCEDURES**

6.1 **Training of personnel**

6.1.1 The personnel need to be properly trained before being able to conduct the procedures independently.

6.1.2 Training of Laboratory Staff Personnel will consist of all the activities that are required to be performed in the stem cell laboratory. Training is imparted in three areas namely

6.1.2.1 Processing of Stem Cells.

6.1.2.2 Instrumentation Operation, Maintenance, Handling and Calibration.

6.1.2.3 General Laboratory activities and Safety.

6.1.3 During the initial training period, Stem Cell units will be processed as part of the Training strategy either by Lab Staff personnel or by the technical specialist of the vendor.

6.1.4 Evaluation of the trainee is done based on the parameters listed in the Internal Stem Cell Laboratory Training Record and/or a training checklist issued by the vendor.

6.1.5 If an external vendor is involved in the initial training, the vendor issuing the training will also provide a training certificate, document a copy of this training certificate along with the internal training record in the Employee file.

6.1.6 As per the Hospital wide policy, no personnel will be allowed to engage in any laboratory activity without a documented training record.

6.1.7 The trainee is explained the entire process and is given opportunity to ask questions.

6.1.8 The trainee will not be allowed to work independently during the Training process.

6.1.9 The Trainee will be required to initially observe the procedure and note down all the steps involved to carry out the process.

6.1.10 The training is followed by an evaluation to determine whether the staff understands the process and is able to independently perform the activities as per the SOP's provided.

6.1.11 The trainee may be allowed to perform all the activities independently only if the trainer determines that the trainee meets all the requirements determined in the Stem Cell Laboratory Training Record.

6.1.12 The minimum score that must be obtained is 3 out of 5. If the score is 2 or below, retraining is done and a fresh training record is prepared.

6.1.13 The entire training activity will be overseen and finally reviewed by the Principal Clinical Scientist before its final approval by the Laboratory Director in-charge of the Blood Bank and Stem Cell section.

6.1.14 After the completing of 6 months, 12 months and thereafter on a yearly basis there will be a competency assessment of the Stem Cell Laboratory staff.

6.1.15 The competency assessment is prepared in accordance with the Hospital wide Policy for competency assessment.

6.1.16 Stem Cell Laboratory staff who fail in the competency assessment is again retrained and an evaluation is made in the Stem Cell Laboratory Training Record.

7. **APPENDICES**

7.1 Stem Cell Laboratory Training Record for Peripheral Blood Stem Cells.

7.2 Staff Competency assessment Record for Peripheral Blood Stem Cells.

8. **ORIGINATING DEPARTMENT/S**

Stem Cell Laboratory

	Name	**Signature**	**Date**
Author			
Review By Study Director			
Q.A. Review			

Fig. 4.3 (continued)

Most SOPs have the following sections:

1. ***Title of an SOP***—The title should be short, to the point, and should highlight the content of the SOP.
2. ***Aim and Purpose/Objective of an SOP***—This section details what the SOP is about and why it is required. It should include statements on the positive implications it aims to have, and how this SOP will improve the Quality and consistency of the process. This SOP has been invariably passed through various stages in the validation process before being recognized in a written document required to be followed by all the parties associated with the process. The purpose of an SOP is to give step-by-step instructions on performing a task so that all the staff members are equally capable without the reliance of an "expert" staff. Some procedures may not be done often, or new staff members may have difficulty performing tasks done by more experienced staff. Thus, SOP acts as a refresher and an educator to the staff. It must be ready "at hand" and be always accessible.
3. ***Scope of an SOP***—The scope section must be the second subtopic in the SOP. It can be an independent section or can be combined with the purpose section in the SOP. First, we need to understand the status of an SOP, and whether it is a new or an old SOP that is being revised. For a Laboratory that focuses on research, the scope involves the area where the SOP is applicable. Areas commonly encountered are process development, experimental procedures, stepwise instructions in the operation and maintenance of equipment, validation procedures for equipment and other procedures that require careful implementation.
   The target audience must be defined. It may be the Manager or a Quality Assurance officer. SOPs can be designed to include several technical details meant to suit several roles based on job responsibilities. Any limitations in the SOP needs to be specified in this section. Next, you must identify the problem the SOP is designed to solve. You must ask yourself, "will this mitigate the risk of failure of the procedure, decrease inaccurate results or prevent accidents?" SOPs are designed to balance risk-benefit modalities.
   The scope of the SOP is to be used as the foundation of the SOP. SOP writers and subject matter experts will need to check if the SOP's objective is being deviated. If there is a deviation in the SOP with respect to the scope, either the SOP needs to be tweaked so that the SOP falls within the scope, or there is a requirement to change the scope to meet the focus of the SOP.
4. ***Responsibility***—This section governs the target audience and the personnel who are required to follow the SOP. Not all staff are required to follow every SOP written in the organization. For example, administrative staff such as Finance and Human Resources (HR) are not required to follow technical SOPs written for the Laboratory. However, HR is required to maintain the Record of Training (ROT) for every staff due to the regulatory requirements and maintenance of records for promotions, assessments, and qualifications.

5. ***Corresponding SOP section***—If an SOP is linked to another SOP, it should be clearly defined here. At times the reader may have to read another SOP as it may have another procedure linked to this protocol. The protocols can be subdivided into various SOPs and this section will give an easy understanding of the associated SOPs to the reader.
6. ***Abbreviations***—Any abbreviation used in the SOP must be written here. SOPs are designed in a way that all personnel should be able to follow it. Not all abbreviations may be known to all staff, hence, it is imperative to document the list of abbreviations.
7. ***Procedure***—This section governs the step-by-step procedure of the process. These steps involve the process from start to finish in a sequential manner. The procedure must be written in present participle tense and not past participle tense. The procedure involves subsections linked in the way of a sequence that combines one subsection to another. The procedure can have subsections such as preparation of reagents, calculations, and Ingredient listings. Any equipment used in the study is listed in a separate subsection.
8. ***Annexures***—List any annexures that may be a part of the SOP. The list of annexures may include forms, work instructions, flowcharts, brochures, or pamphlets that are associated with the SOP. Every document written in the organization has to be a part of the SOP.
9. ***References***—This is the last section in the SOP. List all the reference materials in this section. Reference materials can be published materials, guidelines, websites, manuscripts from journals, or any other form of reference that has aided in writing the SOP.
10. ***Revision History***—This is not a section in the SOP but can be accommodated in the header section or in the section where approvals are granted. The initial or the new SOP can be written as NEW or given a number 0000 (which means that it is a new SOP). The Revision History represents the number of times this SOP is revised. Typically, the SOP is revised every 2 years (which is the lifespan of the SOP) or if any change is required, through a change control (involving technical change or an administrative change). Every change in the SOP (however insignificant) is marked with a number. This is typically designated as 0001. This means that the first change in the SOP has taken place.

4.9 SOP and Work Instructions: What Is the Difference?

SOPs are designated as high-level documents that instruct all employees on the actions that are to be taken. Work instructions specify the particular action in detail. Work instructions can be in the form of a diagrammatic representation or a flowchart. However, mostly they are a step-by-step representation of the process. They are not long, verbose sentences but are expected to be clear, concise, and strictly to the point. Work instructions must be a part within an SOP. As per the ISO 9001, definition of SOP and work instructions, it is mentioned that SOPs are the top layer (Fig. 4.4). They describe which actions are to be taken under a variety of

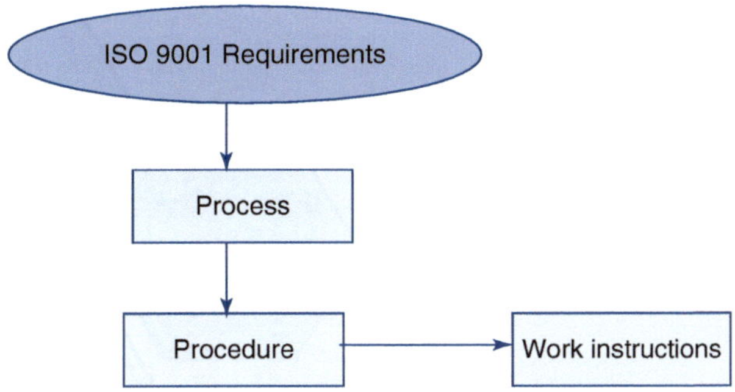

Fig. 4.4 Flowchart of ISO procedures, process, and work instructions

circumstances. However, standard work instructions are the lowest layer. They describe the work to be performed with the lowest possible level of detail. As the name implies, these are instructions to perform a specific piece of work. Some are less than one page or just a list of bullet points. The middle layer and perhaps the most crucial layer, is the process. This can be defined as a measurable objective that consists of input and output activities, and resources. Inputs are requirements that need to be defined while considering the source of the information. This information is required to reach a designed output. Finally, the output is measured by the validation of the end result. This provides insight into the end result.

4.10 Approval and Commissioning of SOPs

SOPs must be signed off prior to their approval for release and implementation. Therefore, the final draft of an SOP must be reviewed, validated, and approved by the authorities described in the quality system of an organization or by an SOP reviewer.

Once approved, an electronic copy of the SOP should be stored in a central server. They must be marked as controlled copies. The hard copies are placed at the location of work. The approval date must be clearly written on the SOP.

4.11 Benefits of SOPs

SOPs are an important part of GLP compliance as it provides a specific directed focus to the end-user or a PhD student. SOPs provide consistency in the methodology, hence this becomes a precursor to reliable results for thesis or a research project. The steps involved in the SOP have been evaluated through a validation process where the recorded results are subjected to statistical analysis or other mathematical interventions. This ensures compliance of the results with established statistical methodologies. PhD scholars must consider SOPs as a fundamental structure in experimental design that provides relevant data with high specificity, consistent quality, and efficiency. Citations of established protocols add value to research in

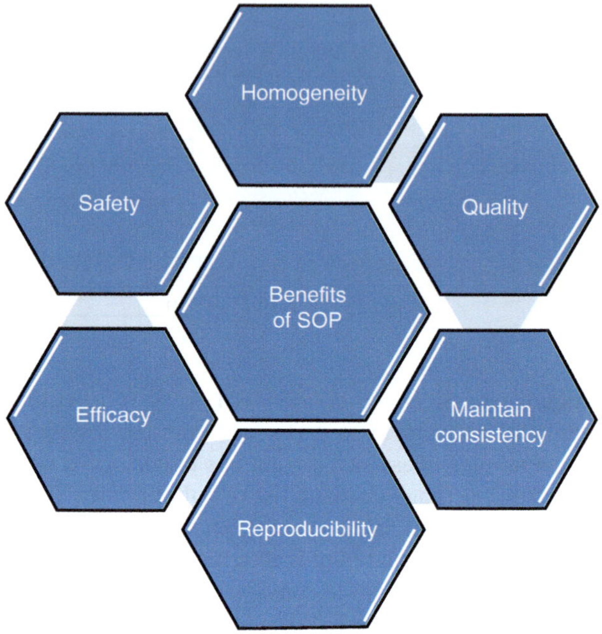

Fig. 4.5 Benefits of an SOP

both clinical as well as nonclinical fields. A well-written SOP prevents erroneous results and thus minimizes wastage of valuable resources and time. Standardization of protocols takes several days to months but this is a precursor to generating data that is reliable, consistent, and above all, accurate. SOPs maintain transparency, consistency, reproducibility, and creditability in the quality system. For a new user, an established SOP helps to carry out the process in an easy, user-friendly manner.

In short, implementation of SOPs can provide the following benefits, summarized in Fig. 4.5:

1. Implementation of SOPs increases the quality of research, maintains homogeneity, and increases reproducibility, resulting in efficacy with minimal errors.
2. SOPs promote consistent outcomes of the results.
3. Implementation of SOPs helps in meeting compliance requirements.
4. SOPs ensure credibility.
5. A well-established SOP helps new hires to get familiar with experiments, thus saving valuable resources in training.
6. SOPs enhance a person's knowledge and skills by providing new thoughts and ideas.

4.12 Implementation of SOPs in PhD or Doctoral Studies

SOPs are not limited to clinical research and pharmaceutical industries. They can be extended to research and other R&D activities voluntarily. SOPs are being stringently implemented in different departments to streamline activities ranging from routine cleaning, sanitation, finance, calibration, documentation, and archival, besides Quality Assurance.

For PhD scholars, SOPs are like the central dogma that provides new opportunities to increase scientific values in nonclinical trials. Implementation of a GLP system, or in particular, SOPs at the doctoral stage (PhD) has its own benefits. The development of SOPs can decrease the time spent by a student on standardization of new procedures developed from routine experimental techniques [31]. Finally, SOPs can save up to a year of time that may be lost in reinventing the wheel. Following an SOP for daily routine activities can help organize daily schedules, which is normally not streamlined in a PhD student's life. In terms of research experimental outcomes and publications, the use of SOPs can add quality, credibility, and reproducibility [32]. Most importantly, exposure to the GLP system and SOPs can help doctoral students adapt to future work environments such as pharmaceutical industries, diagnostic laboratories, and clinical research organizations, where GLP compliance is mandatory, thus giving the students an advantage in employment.

Following SOPs is not without its challenges. It requires continued, long-term commitment from the management and each member of the unit, which can be cumbersome as a laboratory may include students at different stages of their doctoral research. Moreover, since GLP is not mandatory in research laboratories, at the university and doctoral level, it is possible that not all research laboratories follow this strictly. Since research is an interdisciplinary and collaborative field, it may be possible for a laboratory to be GLP-compliant and conducting all procedures as per the defined SOPs; however, common facilities, for example, flow cytometry or even animal husbandry, may not follow such a system. In such a scenario, it would become difficult to control even the simple parameters that can influence an experiment, such as room temperature of an animal house or the calibration routine of equipment's maintained within the common facility. It is here the funding agencies can play a dominant role in compliance. As Coronavirus vaccines are rolled out in Canada, the biggest vaccine manufacturer such as Pfizer-Biotec has recommended a storage temperature for these vaccines. Health Canada has published guidance to this effect. As Pfizer vaccines require storage below −80 °C, research laboratories are called in to aid our colleagues in the clinical setup. This will require a GLP set up and following the SOPs will be mandatory prior to inoculation to the general population. If the PhD scholars are not exposed to following SOPs, it will be difficult to establish a sustained procedure devoid of variations from one province to another, that range from British Columbia to the Maritimes, Tel-Aviv to New York, Auckland to Cape Town.

4.13 Importance of Validation

Validation is considered as verification of data before the generation of an SOP. Data authenticity is the most critical aspect of data in today's scientific world to avoid any falsification. The validation should be double blinded to avoid any bias. This will increase the reliability and reproducibility of data. Today in research, replicability may be affected. So, to maintain the replicability, validation should be implemented. Validation also provides evidence that all work is done with a high degree of assurance and consistency to maintain quality attributes. This ensures that all processes, activities, resources, systems, equipments used in the study are correct and true as self-declared by the user [33].

Validation provides confidence in all fields, especially in pharmaceutical and manufacturing industries, that assure the product quality and consistency with less error and high reproductivity to meet health and regulatory responsibilities. This is also related to auditing of data, which implies organizational maintenance. Validation also rechecks and reconfirms typing error, missing error, sampling error, and incorrect resource data. In 1987, the US Food and Drug Administration (FDA) announced guidelines entitled "GUIDELINES ON GENERAL PRINCIPLES OF PROCESS VALIDATION" [34]. Various studies have shown the importance of validation in research to increase reliability and reproducibility [18, 19].

4.14 Future Directions and Clinical Implications

As regulations evolve regularly, we need to equip our young minds pursuing their PhD degrees to look at regulations as guidelines in their research work. Many Pharma companies have tied up with Research organizations for developing new drugs and vaccines. Thus, PhD candidates need to be equipped in the usage of SOP's that will transition their research from bench to bedside. This is the reason why Regulatory Affairs programs by colleges have gained considerable importance. Regulatory Agencies rely on SOP's for the protocols that are conducted in the laboratories. Evidence of GMP or GLP is ascertained through a robust protocol that follows regulatory guidance. SOP training will provide young students with an opportunity to get trained in SOP writing, which is considered part of the technical writing skill. Companies rely on a good writing acumen while hiring candidates suitable for taking research positions. Within the Clinical area of a Pharmaceutical company, a PhD candidate can work in areas such as R&D, Product Development, Quality, Regulatory, Pharmacovigilance, Clinical Trials, and customer complaints. Having an expertise in SOP writing will give the candidate an expertise in his/her field and thus an opportunity to lead the organization as a Subject Matter Expert (SME) during consultations with major regulatory bodies such as Health Canada or US FDA or EMA. Training in SOPs needs to be inculcated in young minds and this will prove critical in transitioning research from Bench to Bedside.

4.15 Conclusion

An SOP provides the knowledge to complete a specific action. Thus, an SOP is a document that describes the regularly recurring operations relevant to the quality of an investigation or a product or patent. Therefore, the purpose of an SOP is to help carry out the operations correctly and uniformly. It consists of both operational and technical components, which are essential for developing and deploying solutions. SOPs also help the scientists to obtain high-quality results with minimum wastage and promote mutual recognition of results. These guidelines also promote well-planned study followed by performance, data recording, validation, archiving, and data generation, ultimately leading to publication of articles with high consistency in reputed journals and may add value for human welfare. Therefore, in order to make this system a success among PhD students and to reap maximum benefits of the GLP system, it is important to implement these systems at the grassroots level and to involve all the members of the research unit.

References

1. Akyar I. Standard operating procedures (what are they good for?). In: Latest research into quality control, vol. 12. London: IntechOpen; 2012 Dec. p. 367–91.
2. Lindström Gommers L, Mullin T. International conference on harmonization: recent reforms as a driver of global regulatory harmonization and innovation in medical products. Clin Pharmacol Therapeutics. 2019 Apr;105(4):926–31.
3. Robinson K. GLPs and the importance of standard operating procedures. BioPharm Int. 2003 Aug;16(8):38–46.
4. Luthardt FW, Frame LA. Protocol deviations: the importance of communication and documentation. London: Sage; 2020.
5. Schmidt G, Baier D, Hecht A, Herschel M. SOPs in clinical research. Appl Clin Trials. 2013 Jul 1;22(7/8):40.
6. Devine S, Dagher RN, Weiss KD, Santana VM. Good clinical practice and the conduct of clinical studies in pediatric oncology. Pediatr Clin N Am. 2008;55(1):187–209. xi–xii
7. Bhattacharya J, Phill M. Guidance for preparing standard operating procedures (Sops). IOSR J Pharm. 2015;5(1):29–36.
8. De Chadarevian S. Laboratory of molecular biology (LMB). eLS. 2015;15:1–3. https://doi.org/10.1002/9780470015902.a0003409.pub2.
9. Manghani K. Quality assurance: importance of systems and standard operating procedures. Perspect Clin Res. 2011;2(1):34–7.
10. Guideline IH. Integrated addendum to ICH E6 (R1): guideline for good clinical practice E6 (R2). Curr Step. 2015;2:1–60.
11. World Health Organization. Handbook: good laboratory practice (GLP): quality practices for regulated non-clinical research and development. World Health Organization; 2010 Feb 2.
12. Stevens W. Good clinical laboratory practice (GCLP): the need for a hybrid of good laboratory practice and good clinical practice guidelines/standards for medical testing laboratories conducting clinical trials in developing countries. Qual Assur. 2003 Apr 1;10(2):83–9.
13. Bolon B, Baze W, Shilling CJ, Keatley KL, Patrick DJ, Schafer KA. Good laboratory practice in the academic setting: fundamental principles for nonclinical safety assessment and GLP-compliant pathology support when developing innovative biomedical products. ILAR J. 2018 Dec 1;59(1):18–28.
14. Baldeshwiler AM, et al. History of FDA good laboratory practices. Qual Assur J. 2003;7:157–61.
15. OECD. OECD Series on Principles of Good Laboratory Practice and Compliance Monitoring. 1998. http://www.oecd.org/chemicalsafety/testing/oecdseriesonprinciplesofgoodlaboratory-practiceglpandcompliancemonitoring.htm. Accessed 15 Nov 2020.
16. OECD. Principles of good laboratory practice (GLP) and GLP compliance monitoring. In: OECD Chemical safety and overview of good laboratory practice. Paris: OECD; 2020.

17. Peterson O. ISO 9001: the ultimate QMS guide (basics, implementation, ISO templates [Internet]. April 17, 2020. https://www.process.st/iso-9001/
18. Sox HC, Rennie D. Research misconduct, retraction, and cleansing the medical literature: lessons from the Poehlman case. Ann Intern Med. 2006 Apr 18;144(8):609–13.
19. Kaushal MS, Tyagi R, Banik A, Battu MP, Mehra MP, Sharma NK, et al. A unique data validation process by internal and external quality assurance system aimed to combat research malpractice. Int J Sci Res. 2019 Aug;26:8(8).
20. US Food and Drug Administration. Drugs@ FDA: FDA approved drug products. US Food and Drug Administration; 2018.
21. Epa.gov [Internet] U.S. Environmental Protection Agency Report an environmental violation. https://www.epa.gov/. Accessed 6 Dec 2020.
22. Hattemer-Apostel R. Standard operating procedures—a novel perspective. Qual Assur J. 2001;5:207–19.
23. Auditor, What should you expect in any ISO 9001 Internal Auditor Training? ISO 9001 Certification Procedures on July 23, 2018 in ISO 9001 Documents, ISO 9001 Manual, ISO Documents. https://qms9001certificationprocedures.wordpress.com/2018/07/23/iso-9001-2015-internal-auditor-training-and-its-benefits/. Accessed 28 Nov 2020.
24. Fonseca L, Domingues JP. ISO 9001: 2015 edition-management, quality and value. Int J Qual Res. 2017 Mar 14;1(11):149–58.
25. 21 CFR Sec. 211.100 Written procedures; deviations Code of Federal Regulations (annual edition); April 1, 2011.
26. Mine Y, Young D. Regulation of natural health products in Canada. Food Sci Technol Res. 2009;15(5):459–68.
27. Canada.ca. About Natural Health Product Regulation in Canada, Health Canada regulation of natural health products [Internet]. Aug 11, 2016. https://www.canada.ca/en/health-canada/services/drugs-health-products/natural-non-prescription/regulation.html. Accessed 6 Dec 2020.
28. EPA T. Guidance for preparing standard operating procedures (SOPs). J Qual Assur. 2007:1–2.
29. Barbé B, et al. The art of writing and implementing standard operating procedures (SOPs) for laboratories in low-resource settings: review of guidelines and best practices. PLoS Neglected Trop Dis. 10:11.
30. Isaman V, Thelin R. Standard operating procedures (SOPs): reason for, types of, adequacy, approval, and deviations from and revisions to. Qual Assur. 1995 Sep;4(3):167–71.
31. Hollmann S, Frohme M, Endrullat C, Kremer A, D'Elia D, Regierer B, et al. Ten simple rules on how to write a standard operating procedure. PLoS Comput Biol. 2020;16(9):e1008095.
32. Jena GB, Chavan S. Implementation of good laboratory practices (GLP) in basic scientific research: translating the concept beyond regulatory compliance. Regul Toxicol Pharmacol. 2017 Oct 1;89:20–5.
33. Haider SI. Validation standard operating procedures: a step by step guide for achieving compliance in the pharmaceutical, medical device, and biotech industries. Boca Raton, FL: CRC Press; 2006 May 30.
34. Katz P, Campbell C. FDA 2011 process validation guidance: process validation revisited. J GXP Compliance. 2012 Oct 1;16(4):18.

Creating Data Recording Sheets (DRS) in Quality Management System

5

Manjari Rain, Madhava Sai Sivapuram, Deepali Mathur, and K. Sadasivan Pillai

5.1 Introduction

In recent years, the incidences of retraction of scientific articles, even from high-impact journals, have increased [1, 2]. The reasons for retraction include data forgery, non-reproducibility, plagiarism, ethical issues, or scientific error [3]. Thereby, the trust in the published results has declined. In the present era, when research has acquired a fast pace, unknowingly or knowingly referring to unreliable findings delays an essential, most-awaited, and revolutionary scientific discovery. The scientific community requires a system to control the research misconduct by adopting quality measures under Good Lab Practice (GLP) [4]. GLP can be implemented to an independent laboratory or to an entire medical or research institute to produce good quality and reliable data [5]. Journals and grant agencies are adopting various new policies to keep a check on the generation of unreliable data [6]. Recently, Zero effect-Zero defect Youth-Oriented GLP (ZED-YOG) has been proposed for funding agencies to monitor and moderate data generated in projects under the funding agency [7]. ZED-YOG could be instrumental in data scrutiny and validation. However, it is the fundamental duty of the researcher, experimenter, and study director to generate data, which is reliable and reproducible.

M. Rain
Neuroscience Research Lab, Department of Neurology, PGIMER, Chandigarh, India

M. S. Sivapuram
Dr. Pinnamaneni Siddhartha Institute of Medical Sciences and Research Foundation, Chinna-Avutapalli, Andhra Pradesh, India

D. Mathur
Department of Neurology, Apollo Hospital, Bhubaneswar, Odisha, India

K. S. Pillai (✉)
International Institute of Biotechnology and Toxicology, Padappai, Tamil Nadu, India
e-mail: pillaiksp@yahoo.com

A. Anand (ed.), *Quality Assurance Implementation in Research Labs*,
https://doi.org/10.1007/978-981-16-3074-3_5

The target of “reliable and reproducible data” can be achieved by meticulously reporting each step undertaken while performing an experiment. Generally, an experimenter always documents their research findings in a notebook and/or as an electronic copy. However, such documentation is made as per the understanding of the person who is performing the research, i.e., the experimenter. This data may or may not be understandable to a colleague or mentor. Thus, it is obligatory to have a standard data recording system that is easy to maintain, understand and thus provides quality assurance for the experiments and can guarantee reliability and reproducibility of data [8–11]. Each experiment can be documented on a predesigned and standard recording sheet, called a data recording sheet (DRS). The present chapter summarizes how to create a DRS, what information should be included in the DRS, how to record the data in the DRS, and some examples of the templates of DRS.

5.2 Creating a DRS

Before discussing how to create a DRS, it is important to understand the various terminologies around the DRS used in various quality management systems. For example, if we consider the GLP principles, the raw data constitute original laboratory records and documentation, including data directly entered into a computer through an instrument interface. GLP principles define raw data as “the results of original observations and activities in a study which are necessary for the reconstruction of that study.” Similarly, if we consider other quality systems such as National Accreditation Board for Testing and Calibration Laboratories (NABL), the DRS is filled with data. The definition of data in NABL and raw data in GLP practices is more or less the same and is often used interchangeably across different quality systems. In various quality management systems, the DRS is created for recording the results of a study or study-related information that are carried out based on a standardized protocol. Thus, before one generates a DRS, the experiment should be optimized to reach the same output with maximum efficiency for more than three times. Once the protocol has been standardized, the first step is to generate a “Standard operating procedure” (SOP) for the protocol, which must be approved by the mentor in academic research institutions. Before initiating the new experiments, appropriate DRSs should be generated, which are also required to be approved by the mentor. In the next section, we will discuss how to create a new DRS.

5.2.1 DRS in a Research Laboratory Under GLP

Depending on the experiment and its purpose, the DRS may include experimental details, reagent details, sample details, details of the instrument and other materials used in the experiment, and the results of the experiment. Various sections of a typical DRS for MTT assay are given in Figs. 5.1, 5.2, and 5.3. The experimental details should include the volume and concentration of the reagents used per reaction and in total (Fig. 5.1). If the experiment’s duration is more than a day, the experimenter

Restricted Circulation **Photocopying Prohibited**

DATA RECORDING SHEET	Title: MTT Assay					Institute logo
DRS No. AD14-IV05	Student Code:	SOP No.	Copy No.	Experiment No.	Document Controller (Signature/Stamp)	
Experiment Conducted By:	Supervised By:	Date of Issue:	Date of Experiment:			

Experimental Details :

Sr. No.	Experimental Procedure	Date& day	Remarks
1	Plate cells (5000-10000 cells/well)		
2	Serum Starve cells for 12 hours or 24 hours		
3	Washing with PBS (1X)		
4	Stimulate cells with plasma/serum/drug containing media.		
5	Incubate for 24-48 hours		
6	Washing with PBS (1X)		
7	Add 50ul of MTT reagent		
8	Incubate for 3-4 hours		
9	Add 100ul DMSO		
10	Incubate for 15 min. Take absorbance at 595nm		

ABC Institute **XYZ Lab**

Fig. 5.1 A typical DRS for MTT assay: experimental details

should also add the date at which any specific reagent was added into the reaction mixture. Generally, a separate column is kept for adding any remarks or any deviation made from the experiment's approved protocol (Figs. 5.1, 5.2, and 5.3). However, the impact of such deviations on the outcome of the experiment's results should be discussed with the mentor. The experimental details are followed by the reagents' details. In this section, it is necessary to add details of the reagents such as the name of reagent, name of manufacturer, stock concentration, working concentration, catalogue number, batch or lot number, expiry date, and logbook entry details (Fig. 5.2). After entering the details of the reagents, it is equally important to describe the study sample used for the experiment. The type of study sample used, such as cell lysate, plasma or others, source of the sample (sample taken from a control or disease group in case of humans), and treated or untreated sample should be disclosed in the DRS (Fig. 5.2). Other details include volume of the sample used per reaction and any specific remarks, for example, whether the sample was diluted or not.

Lastly, details of the instrument used should also be mentioned in the DRS. This information typically includes name of the manufacturer, catalogue number or model number, batch number, calibration status, and logbook entry details of the use of the instrument. In the end, the experimenter should put his/her signatures in the appropriate column. Following this, the mentor should verify the experiment performed and, upon acceptance, should put his signature in the column assigned (Fig. 5.3).

Restricted Circulation Photocopying Prohibited

DATA RECORDING SHEET	Title : MTT Assay					Institute logo
DRS No.	Student Code:	SOP No.	Copy No.	Experiment No.	Document Controller (Signature/Stamp)	
Experiment Conducted By:	Supervised By:	Date of Issue:	Date of experiment:			

Reagent Details:

Sr. No	Reagent's Name	Manufacturer	Catalogue No.	Batch / Lot No.	Expiry Date: Expired or Fresh	Entered in Log Book	Remarks
1	MTT Reagent						
2	DMSO						
3	PBS						
4	DMEM						

Sample Details

Sr. No.	Sample type (Plasma/ Serum/ CSF) or drug	Disease / drug manufacturer	Percentage of biofluid/ drug used	Expiry or fresh prepared	Remarks

Notes...
....

ABC Institute XYZ Lab

Fig. 5.2 A typical DRS for MTT assay: reagent and sample details

Restricted Circulation Photocopying Prohibited

DATA RECORDING SHEET	Title : MTT Assay					Institute logo
DRS No.	Student Code:	SOP No.	Copy No.	Experiment No.	Document Controller (Signature/Stamp)	
Experiment Conducted By:	Supervised By:	Date of Issue:	Date of experiment:			

Instruments and other materials:

Sl No.	Material/Instrument	Manufacturer	Catalogue No./ Model	Batch / Lot No.	Expiry Date: Expired or Fresh Calibration status	Entered in Log Book	Remarks
1	Autopipettes5ml		.				
2	Autopipettes 10ml						
3	Pipettes & tips : 10µl						
4	Pipettes & tips : 200µl						
5	Pipettes & tips : 1ml						
7	CO_2 Incubator						
8	ELISA Reader (BIORAD)						
9	Weighing balance						

Note:

Approval:	Name	Signature	Date
Author			
Review By Study Director			
Q.A. Review			

ABC Institute XYZ Lab

Fig. 5.3 A typical DRS for MTT assay: instrument and other relevant details

Every page of a DRS should mention the name of the experiment like RT-PCR for gene expression, ELISA, MTT assay, and others. Every page should also have information on the date of issue of DRS, date of experiment, experiment number, name of experimenter, name of supervisor, and a logo of the laboratory or institute (Figs. 5.1, 5.2, and 5.3). It is to be noted that the DRS is created by the experimenter, who has standardized the procedure, and should be approved by the mentor before it is put into regular use of laboratory experiments. In the newly created DRS, the experimenter must ensure that no relevant information has been missed, and unnecessary information has not been included. A well-designed DRS should justify the SOP, and is made in such a way that it is easy to understand and make data entries. A DRS should be concise and informative.

The quality assurance officer or document controller is responsible for issuing the DRS to the experimenter when the experimenter wishes to perform the experiment, and maintains the record of every DRS issued. After an experiment has been performed and details have been filled on the DRS by the experimenter, the mentor should check every detail of the experiment noted on the DRS and the experiment is performed with scientific integrity. Finally, he/she puts their signature on the DRS as an affirmation that the experiment is performed correctly and is accepted as performed. Finally, this filled DRS is returned to the quality assurance officer or document controller for record keeping. The quality assurance officer's responsibility is to see that the DRS is filled in every quality aspect before putting their signature on the DRS. A DRS can be updated on a yearly basis.

5.2.2 DRS in Food and Drug Administration

Food and Drug Administration (FDA) is a federal agency that promotes and protects public health by supervising food safety and drug development. Food products are not limited to packaged unprocessed or processed food for human consumption, but also include animal foods, animal feed, and veterinary products. Drugs include pharmaceutical drugs (medications), vaccines, biopharmaceuticals, blood transfusions, cosmetics, medical devices, and electromagnetic radiation emitting devices [12]. Ready-to-use templates for bioanalytical procedures, which can be used for new drug applications, biologics license applications, and supplements to these applications, are available on the FDA website. These templates are not compulsory but provide guidance to fill the information of bioanalytical procedures of interest [13].

These templates, which are a type of DRS for FDA, also include information on reagents, chemicals, experiments, equipment, and other materials similar to DRS used in academic research. However, the format is different. Here, we are taking an example of a template for pharmacokinetic assessments, which includes three sections for data recording [13]. The first section is for providing "Bioanalytical Method Life Cycle Information," which includes information such as names, expiry date, lot number, serial number, identification number or calibration range for the analyte, reagent, matrix or sample type, and platform or method or equipment, according to applicability [13]. The detailed summary of the method used for pharmacokinetic assessment is filled in the second section, and the third section summarizes any modifications made in the method described in the second section. The third section also includes cross validation results of the modified method. It is to be noted that unlike DRS for academic research, the columns or rows, which are not applicable to the method used for pharmacokinetic assessment can be deleted from the template while reporting [13].

5.2.3 DRS in NABL Accredited Laboratories

NABL is a constituent board of the Quality Council of India whose objective is to provide accreditation to the laboratories across different disciplines (testing laboratories, calibration laboratories, medical laboratories, medical imaging—conformity assessment bodies, proficiency testing providers, and reference material producers) in India and abroad based on the standards set by NABL in accordance with ISO/IEC 17025:2005 and ISO 15189:2012.NABL provides accreditation based on the technical competence and quality of calibration and testing [14]. According to NABL, like GLP, all original observations are required to be maintained in a DRS format by the technical personnel/manager. In NABL, the report (DRS is the report in NABL) is usually termed as the technical report, which includes the date, the personnel responsible for the laboratory activity (Technical Manager), and for checking the data and the results (Quality Manager). As in GLP, the data are recorded as and when they are observed and are identifiable according to the specific task.

A system should always be in place to ensure that the amendments to technical records can be tracked to previous versions or original observations of these records. An ISO 17025 NABL accredited facility should always monitor its performance by comparing its results with other ISO 17025 NABL accredited laboratories. An ISO 17025 NABL test report is not an elaborately written report like a GLP study report, and the findings are usually reported in a tabular form in a NABL test report. A typical NABL test report of a product "xyz" tested against antimicrobial property is given in Table 5.1.

Usually, NABL test is carried out using a standard test method and the method used for the testing is mentioned in the report. There is no need to describe the test method in detail in the NABL test report. The result in these reports is given as Pass/Fail or Complies/Does not comply. These test reports are signed by the technical manager (the terminology study director/experimenter/researcher is not used in NABL ISO 17025 system) and quality manager.

5.2.4 DRS for Toxicity Test

Toxicity testing is usually done on experimental animals and the purpose of doing a toxicity test is to determine the extent of dose and the potential hazards of a test substance among these experimental animals before administrating them into humans for clinical trials [15]. It enables us to understand more about the substance and helps create a dose–response curve, mechanism of action, potential adverse effects, and the safety of the substances administered [15–17].

An example of the DRS used for toxicity testing in the animals is given in Table 5.2. In this DRS, the species, route of administration of the substance,

Table 5.1 An example of antimicrobial property of product xyz

Product details						
Product ID			Batch/lot no.			
Name of the product			Quantity received			
Sample product			Test method/ specification		IP 2018	
Name of microorganism	Colony Forming Unit (CFU) for contact time				Suspension strength	Result
	0 min	01 min	03 min	05 min		
Staphylococcus aureus	TNTC	TNTC	TNTC	TNTC	1.4×10^6 cfu/ml	Fail
Pseudomonas aeruginosa	TNTC	TNTC	TNTC	TNTC	1.6×10^6 cfu/ml	Fail
Candida albicans	TNTC	TNTC	TNTC	TNTC	1.0×10^5 cfu/ml	Fail
Signature Technical Manager				Signature Quality Manager		

TNTC, too numerous to count; cfu, colony forming units

Table 5.2 An example of dosing record of animals

Format no.												
Version No.												
Study no.			**Group:**			**Dose:**			**Weighing balance/ Micropipette ID:**			
Species:			**Route of administration:**						**Vehicle:**			
Day →			1			2			3			
Date →												
Cage no	Animal No.	Sex	Body weight (g /kg)	Dose (mg/kg or ml/kg)	Dose Vol.[a](ml)	Body weight (g /kg)	Dose (mg/kg or ml/kg)	Dose Vol.[a](ml)	Body weight (g / kg)	Dose (mg/kg or ml/kg)	Dose Vol. [a](ml)	
Sign and Date												
[a]Dose volume (in the case of oral route of administration) = Animal body weight(g) × 10 (ml)/1000 g (Note-In this case the volume of dose administered is 10 ml/kg body weight.)												

[a]Dose volume (in the case of oral route of administration) = Animal body weight(g) × 10 (ml)/1000 g
(Note: In this case the volume of dose administered is 10 ml/kg body weight)

bodyweight of the animal (g or kg), and dose volume (ml) are recorded apart from the dose (mg or kg or ml/kg). In repeated dose administration studies, toxicity testing is done multiple times on a single experimental animal to establish the dose-response curve and hence, multiple rows of days are given. At the end of the DRS, the signature of the person performing the experiment and the date should always be added.

5.3 Recording Data in DRS

In DRS, the data should be recorded using a blue ballpoint pen with indelible ink as and when the activity is performed. Uniformity needs to be maintained across all the data records like AM and PM or the 24-h format for recording the time, recording of the date in a particular format like following the date, month and year or the month, date, and year format. The date and time of the experiment should be noted down accurately. No blank spaces must be present in the DRS sheets, wherever not applicable, use N/A. The signature and the date must be filled on the same day when the entry is made, and the unused portion of the page must be strike down with a line, preferably a diagonal one along with the signature and date. The observations recorded in the DRS sheet must be accurate and appropriate along with legibility. Special care must be taken while recording the unit of the measurements wherever applicable.

It is always possible for errors to occur while collecting the data or there might be corrections in the data while/after performing the experiment, so a clear audit trail is needed to explain the reason for the change in the data. While correcting the data, it must be noted that correction fluid or erasing of data must not be done. Instead, a separate line is drawn over the original entry and then the correct entry with dated signature or initial is added. After the corrected entry is made, the error is encircled to differentiate it from the corrected entry and the other entries in the DRS. Try to use an error code that can explain the reason for the change in the entry or the error in the data entry in the DRS, as close to the corrected entry as possible. If space is a problem, then put these error codes as a note in the form of a table.

Some of the error codes with abbreviations are: Changed for greater clarity (CC), Calculation error (CE), Miscount (MS), Inadvertently not signed and dated at the time of observation (ND) (this particular error is considered as a serious observation by the auditors), Out of proper sequence (OS), Recording error (RE), Sampling error (SE), Spelling error (SR), Wrong dosing (WD), Wrong date (WE), Inadvertently recorded in wrong location (WL), and Write over (WO).

The personnel recording the data in the DRS should be extremely careful and always make a note of significant figures, especially for the arithmetic operations. Significant figures are the numbers that reflect any measurement, which is considered as the correct value within an implied error limit. The whole numbers (digits between 1 and 9) are always considered significant. When it comes to "0", it is significant if present in between whole numbers irrespective of the decimal point; if a "0" is present on the right side of any whole number, it may or may not be

Table 5.3 Examples of significant figures

Value	Unit	No. of significant figures
31.34	cm	4
23.03	cm	4
0.25	m	2
0.013	m	3
2.0064	g	5
33.000	kg	2
320.000	kg	6

The significant figures are underlined

significant; if the "0" is present to locate a decimal point, then it is significant. Table 5.3 shows a few examples of the significant figures to clarify this confusion. When rounding off the decimal number, a few rules need to be followed. If the last number is more than "5", then "1" is added to the adjacent number whereas if the last number is less than "5", then "0" is added to the adjacent number. If the last number is "5", then "1" is added if the adjacent number is odd, and "0" is added if the adjacent number is even.

Sometimes, a deviation from the SOP, or the study protocol can occur while recording data in DRS. If any such deviation happens, the reason for the deviation must be recorded and reported to the mentor. The DRS sheets can be audited anytime by the quality assurance officer.

5.4 Electronic Recording of Data and eDRS

With the advent of computational technology, automation systems, information technology, and cloud computing, recording of the data can also be done via web applications that can be accessed via browsers or phone applications on phones or tablets. Hence, specific care must be taken to include the date, study/experiment number, sample identity/number, instrument details and parameters, digital signature of the personnel recording the data. It should be noted that the data and observations generated by the machine and electronic media are distinguished by date and maintained in separate folders. These data or observations are in a specific format and thus, are defined as electronic DRS or eDRS. While using these computerized DRS, the personnel and the study director are responsible for 100% entry of the data and data check. Raw data are in eDRS in the form of electronic storage media or computer/instrument printouts. Recent technology has led to the development of equipment's that generates eDRS that can be used directly for data analysis. Generally, the equipment-generated DRS are in different formats depending on the instrument. These files have extensions such as .eds, .map, .fam, .bim, which can be converted or opened in Microsoft Excel or Microsoft Notepad. It is to be noted that alterations cannot be made in the original data of eDRS with specific extensions. Changes can only be made during the analysis. System design should provide a full audit trail to show all changes to raw data without obscuring the original data. Persons who make changes to the raw data should put the time, date, and electronic signature. Reasons for changes should also be provided. Any manually entered data should be clearly identified and retained.

A manual backup procedure and an alternate data capture procedure should be in place to minimize the risk of any data loss in the event of system failure. Although cloud computing helps with the virtual backup, having both the manual and the virtual backup will secure the data and help in data restoration in case of data loss due to system failure. When the data and eDRS stored in a system are moved to another system, it should be ensured that exact copy of the data and eDRS are migrated to the new system.

Security procedures should be in place for the prevention of corruption of data, unauthorized modification of data, and for prevention of unauthorized access. Access to electronic data and eDRS must be with a unique user identity and should be password protected. Only authorized personnel should have access to the hardware, peripheral components, or electronic storage media. The introduction of data and software from an external source should be controlled by the computer system software and specific security routines.

In an academic research laboratory that follows GLP, all personnel should be aware of the procedures and system features to provide appropriate security and must be aware of the consequences of security breaches. It is essential and important to make backup copies of all software and raw data. The backup copy is also retained as an original document.

5.5 Coding, Indexing, and Location of DRS

Several SOPs and DRS are followed in a quality management system. Hence, these need to be master coded by the quality assurance officer. The master code can be of any format, such as numerical or a mixture of numeric and alphabets, depending on the quality management system. An example of master coding is displayed in Fig. 5.4. Generally, an alphabetic code indicating the type of DRS can be used for coding; some of the examples are BE for biochemical estimations, MB for Molecular Biology, IT for Immuno-technology, AN for Animal study, NP for Neuropsychology, IV for In vitro experiments, and others. Some of the routine activities, such as preparation of buffers, autoclaving, and blood sample collection fall under the general criteria and may use GN (General) for coding.

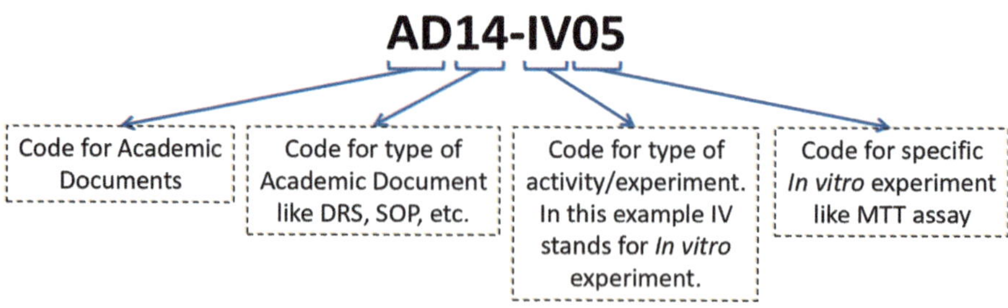

Fig. 5.4 An example for Master coding of DRS

When required by the experimenter, DRS can be issued under their name by the quality assurance officer. The quality assurance officer makes an entry regarding which DRS was issued to the experimenter. The used DRS is returned to the quality assurance officer, who keeps the DRS in the experimenter's file. All DRS are neatly indexed with date of issue, date of return, signature of the experimenter at both instances and, signature of the quality assurance officer. An example of an issue log sheet is shown in

Restricted Circulation **Photocopying Prohibited**

ISSUE LOG: Data Record Sheet

Institute logo

ITEM:AD14				
Location:				
DRS No.	**Edition No.**	**Effective Date**	**Review Date**	**Document Controller (Signature/Stamp)**
Copy No.	**Date of Issue with Signature**	**Date of receipt with Signature**		

Sr. No.	Issue date	Name of the student	Name of data recording sheet	Qty	Student code	Return date	Sign	Remarks

Approvals:

	Name	Signature	Date
Author and In-life Observer			
Q.A. Review			
Management Approval			

ABC Institute AD14-01 **XYZ Lab**

Fig. 5.5 An example of Issue log sheet for DRS

Fig. 5.5. A used DRS is not issued to another experimenter. If required, the other experimenter can refer to the used DRS in presence of quality assurance officer or mentor.

All the DRS and eDRS should be archived under a project or in the name of a particular person, after completion of the work. Both, the hardcopy and the softcopy of DRS are archived the way other types of data are archived. Kindly refer to Chap. 10 for details on archiving. Procedures should be in place to ensure the data's long-term integrity and continuous readability (producing hard copy printouts, copying data to another system). Electronically stored data cannot be destroyed without management authorization and proper documentation. Other data held in support of computerized systems, such as source code and development, validation, operation, maintenance, and monitoring records, should be held for at least as long as study records associated with these systems.

5.6 Significance of Record Keeping in Scientific Research

Science is based on accumulation of facts and evidence. To trust those facts, it is crucial to keep a good record of scientific investigations. The best way is to pen down all necessary steps a researcher/experimenter is following while performing the experiment at that particular time. If one does not note them down, it becomes difficult for other researchers to rely upon the findings and to validate if they want to repeat it. If another researcher wishes to perform the same experiment, the research should be described in sufficient detail so that they can easily perform it. Furthermore, it is the liability of each member of the research group to maintain their research records. To maintain good laboratory records, one should follow certain rules. For instance, each member of the group involved in a scientific experiment should possess a laboratory notebook in which they can write down the protocol they are following, daily laboratory activity, calculations related to the experiment, making notes of important information on a daily basis, so that they can take a look at it whenever required. This data can be recorded in a more pertinent way for others to understand, reanalyze and interpret the findings in the form of DRS, so that the data is auditable and can be backtracked. Thus, a unique validation of the generated data can be carried out at any time [18]. There are several reasons as to why an experimenter should keep a good scientific record. These are discussed below:

1. Good record keeping is indispensable for data analysis, publication, peer review, collaboration, and other research activities. If one has maintained good record keeping, it is easier for an experimenter to view and reanalyze their data whenever required, publish their work, discuss with their peers, redraft, and amend the research work planned for the future and collaborate with other researchers. After submitting the manuscript to a journal, if a reviewer and/or editor asks for supplementary material or supporting data, one should be able to track and show them the data to support their findings. There is also a possibility that after the work is published in a scientific journal, one is asked to deposit their data in a

data repository and share it with the team members who want to perform the same research again or assess the work thoroughly.

2. Another reason why the experimenters must maintain records is that many research institutions and hospitals where the work is being carried out may ask for records and other related documents after the work is published. There are certain institutional guidelines, and in order to meet them and ensure excellence for the conduct of good science, they may ask for it later. Hence, experimenters must be ready with their records even after publication.
3. Good record keeping is required to reinforce intellectual property rights. If an experimenter has filed a patent for their research or involves intellectual property, then they can show his/her records at any time to support their application if they have maintained it.
4. Good record keeping can also safeguard against fallacious claims from other researchers for research misconduct. If another experimenter fails to perform the same research already published in a journal, there are chances that they can put allegations against the researcher for their findings not being supported by evidence. This may happen if the research/experiment has not been described in sufficient detail, or the research paper lacks important facts to allow the other experimenter to repeat the work.

   During the past decade, thousands of papers have been retracted from various international journals. Although some papers were retracted due to calculation errors or the other errors made which were genuine mistakes, but most of them were retracted because of various factors, among which data falsification, data duplication has played a major role [19]. One such controversy happened a decade ago. In 2009, a German anesthesiologist faced retraction of almost 96 articles among the 98 published articles. The articles were on intravenous solutions containing hetastarch or hydroxyethyl starch, which are used to stabilize blood pressure during and after surgery or trauma [1]. The reason for the retraction was the huge data fabrication and misconduct, ignoring the ethics. The most recent data infringement during the pandemic of COVID-19 is data falsification regarding the use of hydroxychloroquine drug among COVID-19 patients, which resulted in retrieval of papers from *Lancet* and *NEJM* journals, and wastage of hundreds and thousands of dollars on the clinical trials that were started across the world [20, 21]. The company involved in this falsification was Surgisphere. Using the DRS, the data infringement, falsification, or duplication can be minimized. DRS are helpful in showing the integrity and validity of the data collected. Hence, it is vital to keep a good record of what you do in the laboratory, so that you do not face any fabrication or falsification charges.
5. Lastly, good record keeping plays a cardinal role in the management of human subjects. Documentation related to research involving patient samples and healthy controls must be recorded. It is important to mention here that human samples are really precious, and in order to conduct research using them, the researchers/experimenters have to get it approved by the institutional ethical

committee whose records and informed consents should be readily accessible upon request.

5.7 Future Directions and Clinical Implications

Manual recording of the DRS is being replaced by the electronic DRS and the software is currently under development for electronic data recording. This will facilitate record keeping and management of archived data. However, robust measures should be taken to avoid data corruption, and deletion of electronic DRS. Use of DRS in research lab is in its initial phases. Some countries and institutes follow it religiously. However, global implementation of DRS is essential to increase reliability and reproducibility of data for effective and economical translation, thereby increasing the probability of discoveries and inventions. DRS is essential in clinical research as it is in experimental research, for proper record of raw data in a timely manner. In clinical trials, all necessary information related to recruitment of volunteers should be as per the regulatory guidelines and recorded in the DRS. The quantity and time of the drug administrated or type of intervention are also recorded in DRS. Similarly, clinical observations made on the volunteers are entered in appropriately designed DRS. This DRS is not only for record keeping but also to enable audit trails.

Acknowledgment We acknowledge Dr. Akshay Anand for providing examples of DRS.

References

1. Brainard J, You J. What a massive database of retracted papers reveals about science publishing's 'death penalty'. Science. 2018;25(1):1–5.
2. Piller C, Servick K. Two elite medical journals retract coronavirus papers over data integrity questions. Science. 2020;4(10):1126.
3. Steen RG. Retractions in the scientific literature: is the incidence of research fraud increasing? J Med Ethics. 2011;37(4):249–53.
4. Kumar S, Mehra P, Anand A. Policy research into quality assessment of published data from medical institutes can increase the authenticity of translation. Ann Neurosci. 2020;27(2):45–6.
5. Anand A, Tyagi R, Kaur P. Policy research for assessment of quality assurance practices in skill development of doctoral programs in medical institutes. Ann Neurosci. 2017;24(3):134.
6. Ten Cate O, Brewster D, Cruess R, Calman K, Rogers W, Supe A, et al. Research fraud and its combat: what can a journal do? Med Educ. 2013;47(7):638–40.
7. Tyagi R, Anand A. Development and implementation of ZED-YOG quality module: Niyantrita Madhumeha Bharata skill development initiatives. Ann Neurosci. 2019;26(1):37–44.
8. Fisher DL. Data, documentation, and decision tables. Commun ACM. 1966;9(1):26–31.
9. Blank G, Rasmussen KB. The data documentation initiative: the value and significance of a worldwide standard. Soc Sci Comput Rev. 2004;22(3):307–18.
10. Göpferich S. Data documentation and data accessibility in translation process research. Translator. 2010;16(1):93–124.
11. Vardigan M, Heus P, Thomas W. Data documentation initiative: toward a standard for the social sciences. Int J Digit Curation. 2008;3(1):107–13.

12. US Food and Drug Administration [Internet]. https://www.fda.gov/. Accessed 07 Jan 2021.
13. U.S. Department of Health and Human Services, Food and Drug Administration, Center for Drug Evaluation and Research (CDER). Bioanalytical Methods Templates. Guidance for Industry Technical Specifications Document. 2019. https://www.fda.gov/media/131425/download. Accessed 28 Nov 2020.
14. NABL. Nabl India [Internet]. 2020. https://nabl-india.org/. Accessed 29 Nov 2020.
15. Bhattacharya S, Zhang Q, Carmichael PL, Boekelheide K, Andersen ME. Toxicity testing in the 21 century: defining new risk assessment approaches based on perturbation of intracellular toxicity pathways. PLoS One. 2011;6(6):e20887.
16. Parasuraman S. Toxicological screening. J Pharmacol Pharmacother. 2011;2(2):74–9.
17. Arome D, Chinedu E. The importance of toxicity testing. J Pharm BioSci. 2013;4:146–8.
18. Kaushal MS, Tyagi R, Banik A, Battu MP, Mehra MP, Sharma NK, et al. A unique data validation process by internal and external quality assurance system aimed to combat research malpractice. Int J Sci Res. 2019;8(8):5–9.
19. Trikalinos NA, Evangelou E, Ioannidis JP. Falsified papers in high-impact journals were slow to retract and indistinguishable from non fraudulent papers. J Clin Epidemiol. 2008;61(5):464–70.
20. Davey M, Kirchgaessner S, Boseley S. Surgisphere: governments and WHO changed Covid-19 policy based on suspect data from tiny US company [Internet]. The Guardian. Guardian News and Media; 2020. https://www.theguardian.com/world/2020/jun/03/covid-19-surgisphere-who-world-health-organization-hydroxychloroquine. Accessed 26 Nov 2020.
21. The Lancet Editors. Expression of concern: hydroxychloroquine or chloroquine with or without a macrolide for treatment of COVID-19: a multinational registry analysis. Lancet (London, England). 2020;395(10240):e102.

The Value of Master Schedules in Benchmarking Research Productivity

6

Pranay Mahajan, Shweta Modgil, and Vipin Koushal

6.1 Introduction

Research is the most enchanting form of science where one can very easily get overwhelmed or carried away from the core objectives. Even though the main project may have been well defined with goals and objectives having a flawless methodology and an insight about expected outcomes, the most challenging part is the "execution of the plan." When a researcher actually gets down to the work, the likelihood of going off track and working on parallel tangential experiments is very high. The beauty of research lies in the fact that one may end up with entirely different results than expected in the beginning and such observations are always welcomed. However, a number of undesirable subjective factors like indolence, ignorance, complacency, procrastination, negligence, apathy, etc. may hamper the efficiency expected out of researchers involved in any research project. Similarly, organization and research setup specific factors like leadership, work culture, workload, adherence to standard procedures and protocols, monitoring techniques, reporting and feedback, contingency measures, defining goals and objectives, etc. also influence the efficiency and reliability of research activities. Be it an individual

P. Mahajan
Department of Hospital Administration, Post Graduate Institute of Medical Education and Research, Chandigarh, India

S. Modgil
Emory Eye Center, School of Medicine, Emory University, Atlanta, GA, USA

V. Koushal (✉)
Department of Hospital Administration, Post Graduate Institute of Medical Education and Research, Chandigarh, India

Department of Biostatistics, Post Graduate Institute of Medical Education and Research, Chandigarh, India
e-mail: koushal.vipin@pgimer.edu.in

A. Anand (ed.), *Quality Assurance Implementation in Research Labs*,
https://doi.org/10.1007/978-981-16-3074-3_6

research project or larger organizational programs encompassing multiple projects, accomplishing the objectives within a set timeframe in a time-bound manner critically determines the productivity of such projects. Any research work involves huge investments in terms of man, material, and money, and the results are expected to be meaningful, reliable, and dependable. This necessitates a high level of efficiency in the research productivity and therefore proper planning and scheduling of all related activities become vital. This can be achieved in any research setup through well-crafted "Master Schedules". Master scheduling ensures that the planned research project is affected in a systematic manner within set timeframes and assures quality in work. Master Schedules of different projects synced together also assures efficiency in overall programs being carried out by the research organization.

When we talk about the significance of master scheduling in research, factors like time constraints linked to the projects in hand, strict implementation and scrutiny of funded projects, coupled with mandated submission of various reports for the project renewal, make the scheduling of plans almost indispensable for productive research. Tracking of ongoing projects has become crucial in recent years. In fact, most of the funding agencies ask for a timeline of project beforehand, where objectives are broken down into achievable targets to ensure the feasibility of project completion in a given timeframe. According to the Organization for Economic Cooperation and Development (OECD) Principles of Good Laboratory Practice (GLP), Master Schedule is "a compilation of information to assist in the assessment of workload and for the tracking of studies at a test facility" [1].

6.2 Master Schedule

A Master Schedule is *an integration of all the schedules defined for achieving various feasibly planned objectives of the project and elucidates timeline and relationship between all the activities. It defines each milestone of the project and specifies its date along with the time required to achieve each objective.*

Master Schedule is an operational management and quality assurance tool which gives a logical timeline to various planned activities in the Master Plan of any research project. It is a well-planned and feasible integration of all these activities on a time-scale taking into consideration the relationship between different activities as well as the resource allocation aspects. For example, if two different activities in a project require the same resources but are independent of each other and need not be taken up at the same time, the two would be accommodated on different time periods on the timeline of the master schedule. Master schedules also provide the breakup of work between different teams/researchers and their supposed schedules of work.

There is no stiff format that a master schedule needs to adopt; its formation and extent are flexible as per the requirements and resources of the research project or organization. However, once finalized, it is a rigid schedule to be adhered to. It sets the milestones to be achieved at specified times in the journey of efficiently productive research. It helps one to break down a big task into deliverables in smaller time frames of days and months. For example, a researcher can divide his 1-month tasks either broadly into 4 weeks or even micromanage on a daily basis taking cues from the master schedule. Basically, it gives highlights of project activities on a daily, monthly, and yearly basis and helps keep a track of the progress of research work.

Master schedules can be formulated for each individual project as well as one for the whole of the projects being undertaken in an organization. A glance at the master schedule of entire studies ongoing in the test facility can help the management to contemplate the workload of the facility. It helps them track the overall progress of different ongoing projects of the organization and thereby aids in appropriate resource allocation and corrective steps wherever required. Besides, helping the quality assurance specialist (QA) and the organizational management in GLP-related inspections and assessments, it spares research personnel from the hassle of setting their priorities each day. One of the biggest challenges for a researcher at the start of her day is to choose a task from a handful of experiments, to begin with. Most of the time, researchers waste their most productive time in deciding which experiment to start. Master schedule comes handy in this situation where one does not waste time and energy in scrolling from the wishlist of all her experiments; instead, she is very clear in her mind what experiment she should put her energy into. It also saves them from 'Monday Morning Syndrome' where lack of planning may affect the project due to unavailable resources.

6.2.1 Formative Elements of a Master Schedule and Its Formation

As discussed earlier, the Master Schedule need not follow a set format and can be flexibly devised as per the requirements of the project and programs. However, it invariably has certain essential formative elements which must be well understood by the readers.

A Master Schedule is unvaryingly created based upon two things:

1. A Master Plan
2. Detailed Work Schedules

Before we proceed, just remember that creating a Master Schedule involves a "Bottom-up Approach." Let us understand this. Any research project has a master "plan" (commonly referred to as a research protocol) which provides details about the aim, objectives, methodology, and required resources. For productive research work, all the activities must always be carefully planned right from the beginning of the work, starting from its commencement till its results and meaningful dispersal of the results to the scientific community. This is done by taking inputs from all stakeholders (investigators and others) involved or expected to be involved in the work in due course of time. All stakeholders have their piece of work and responsibilities toward the work. There may be a Director/Chief/Principal Investigator of the project and single or multiple teams with team leads. The teams (or individuals as the case may be) are asked to submit a schedule for the planned activities in their domain, commonly referred to as "Detailed Work Schedule (DWS)." A DWS includes a detailed timeline for all the milestones to be achieved by the team/individual members and details of the resources required with a specific time of their need in the study. All the DWSs from various teams/individuals when submitted to the project leader enables him to finally create a "Master Schedule" of activities for the project. This Master Schedule is developed by incorporating all the DWSs in a comprehensive manner, integrating their timelines and resources on a meaningful timescale. It lists all the activities at different levels of the project, their interrelationships and relation to all milestones and outputs of the project. And we must have understood by now why Master Scheduling is said to be a "bottom-up approach."

To put it in simple words, for a project to be efficiently executed, it is first thoroughly *planned* (Master Plan) and then a *schedule* (Master Schedule) is assigned for timely completion of all its activities. Peter Turla has aptly said; "*A plan is what, a schedule is when. It takes both a plan and a schedule to get things done*."

Following are some key points to remember while formulating a Master Schedule:

- It must contain specifics of every milestone in the research project and provide for its date.
- It must document all the activities and provide interrelationships amongst them.
- It must illustrate the time allocated for achieving different objectives of the research work.
- It must specify the expected dates of various outcomes.
- Highest possible degree of precision must be ensured in formulating Master Plan and DWSs as the effectiveness of Master Schedule primarily depends upon the quality and accuracy of information derived from these two sources.
- The Master Plan must clearly state the scope and objectives of the work and appropriately describe the organization, resources, and training requirements for the project.
- Master Plan must include the details of every significant activity in the project and provide for "Work Breakdown Structure (WBS)" on the basis of which DWSs are formulated.
- Those persons who would actually be doing an activity must be involved in formulating the schedule (DWS) for that activity.
- DWSs should be formulated for each and every activity of the project and must provide an accurate estimate of required time and resources.
- Time-period and resource allocation for all the activities in the final Master Schedule must be adequately "cushioned" so that minor delays do not affect the overall progress of the project. This becomes especially important keeping in mind the fact that a finalized Master Schedule is quite a rigid time schedule.
- Risk assessment in relation to each activity must be done thoroughly in the planning phase and master schedule must include adequate contingency cushioning for the same.

6.2.2 Before Preparing a Master Schedule

Now that we understand if a Master schedule is prepared with thoughtful planning, it helps one to conduct research activities smoothly in lab and it leads to quality data production. Certain things should be kept in mind before starting to prepare the master schedule. These include:

1. **Discussion with QA/Study Director:**
   Before committing to the DWSs of project activities, it is always a good decision to have a discussion with the study director (in case the study director and research personnel are different entities). A thorough discussion about the expectation of the study director, tasks that require immediate attention and feasibility of tasks in the given timeframe helps to carve out a schedule that will yield good quality data at the end. Discussion beforehand spares the researcher from the hassle of last moment hitches in the experiment.
2. **Standard Operating Procedures (SOPs):**
   The Master Schedule system to be followed by a facility must be methodically described in an SOP. SOPs form a necessary prerequisite for GLP. There must be an SOP in place which provides for set procedures to be followed while devising and executing the Master Schedule(s) in the facility. In brief, SOP should include all the information in a step-wise manner for the ease of a person who can use it as a reference to generate Master Schedule in the future. It elaborates the procedures for making, documenting, and archiving of master schedule as per defined format. It should provide information regarding the format and content of master schedule. What to include in it and how (hand filled/printed) and when it should be provided to QA (e.g., last week of the previous month or 1st working day of the month) can be elaborated. It should further contain the specifics regarding who is responsible to create, manage and evaluate the Master Schedule. Information related to how changes can be made and how frequently can it be revised should also be mentioned. The SOP for master schedule can elaborate on the font, word size, and contents of the Master Schedule.
3. **Do not become overambitious about setting unrealistic goals:**
   Well-thought and planned master schedule is the key to quality data in research. Master schedule should be made keeping all the aspects of research in mind. While formulating the DWSs by the researchers, underestimation of their own potential and writing vague schedules results in too less work done due to low commitment and non-planning and would have an adverse effect on the Master Schedule of the project. On the other hand, overambition leaves one with the setting of unrealistic goals. The latter may lead to lesser work accomplished in the devoted time period and would also affect the quality of work. In addition, committing to too much work leads to anxiety. Therefore, planning a master schedule is a task that requires a clear and concise picture in the mind about the feasibility of the schedules submitted by researchers. To assure achievable schedules being incorporated in the Master Schedule, group discussions must be held between team leads, its members, and the management including the project

director prior to submission of finalized DWS. Similarly, the Master Schedule must also be formulated and finalized after thorough discussion with all stakeholders of the project.

4. **What is a rescue or backup plan if you failed to keep up with the schedule?**
   Good lab practices module advocates an important aspect related to research activities, i.e., backup plan or a Contingency Plan. For every Plan-A, there should be a replaceable Plan-B. For a given master schedule, keeping alternative options to mitigate the effects of avoidable and unavoidable exigencies is always a better choice. Rescue plan saves the system from strain and researcher from stress related to failure. What if one fails to keep up with the master schedule? Has it been planned in a way that he/she can still be able to work it out over the remaining time period by working for some extra time each day or on weekends? What if the tasks scheduled for a researcher over a period of time could not be accomplished due to any reason, have the flexibility of time and resources been planned in the master schedule which may be diverted to the lagging activities to catch up with the scheduled pace of the project? Master Schedule must therefore have adequate "cushioning" in terms of time as well as resources to meet all such exigencies. For example, a researcher falls sick for a prolonged period and his/her particular activities are hampered, there must be a planned backup of dully skilled human resources to cover up this lag, so that the overall pace of the project does not get hampered. In the case of interrelated activities where one activity is dependent on the pace or completion of another activity, due caution must be exercised to ensure adequate cushioning being provided in the Master Schedule so that delays in the preceding one do not hamper the succeeding one. Activities critical to the progress of a project must be kept on top priority in the Master Schedule with adequate contingency measures and strict monitoring. Management tools like PERT (Program Evaluation and Review Technique) and CPM (Critical Path Method) come in handy in such situations. These would be discussed in later parts of this chapter.

5. **Integration of Master Schedules and harmonized scheduling:**
   We have talked about Master Schedules from both perspectives viz. for a specific project and also for the whole facility. In case of later, when the facility is running various projects simultaneously, the top management and director/chief of the facility must devise a Master Schedule of all the projects in toto, taking into account the critical milestones of all projects running concurrently. Besides helping the management in thoughtful comprehensive monitoring of total programs of the facility for the overall efficiency of the research facility, it also helps them in steering the resources toward lagging projects and in scenarios of contingency nature. For example, a particular project "A" utilizes an electricity-based equipment in its experiments. There is an unexpected power failure for 3 days and project "A" (*as evident from its Master Schedule*) has already consumed its "cushioning" capacity and would further lead to an undesirable delay in the whole project. Another project "B" utilizes a non-electricity-based equipment for the same experiments and can produce similar results as being produced by the electricity-based equipment of project "A." A glance at the Master

Schedule of project "B" also confirms that there is adequate "cushioning" time available in that project related to the experiment utilizing this equipment. Now the "Master Schedule of the whole facility" would help management in prompt identification of the scenario in project "B" and after verification of feasibility (with stakeholders of project "B") to temporarily divert the resource to project "A," they can efficiently keep it going.

6.2.3 Preparing the Master Schedule (Format and Contents)

Responsibilities for generation, maintenance, and archiving of master schedule should be defined at the beginning of the research work. The QA is given the responsibility for maintenance and archiving of the master schedule sheets but the onus of its generation is not necessarily on him [2]. The master schedule can be generated by the study director or research personnel. In the case of the Facility Master Schedule, the same may be generated by the Chief of the facility/Operational Chief or a person designated on their behalf. Sample formats for Master Schedules for an individual project and for the whole facility have been provided in Figs. 6.1 and 6.2. Also, an example of DWS has been depicted in Fig. 6.3.

As discussed earlier, the format of the Master schedule is generally adopted by individual lab as per their own needs [3]. It may be generated through a computer in a typed and printed form and the copies provided to QA and management; or it may be hand filled in the prescribed format. Generally, the **content of MS is given more importance than the format**. Contents can also vary from lab to lab and it depends

MASTER SCHEDULE Project Code : XXXXXX			Data Controller (Signature/Stamp)	Organisation LOGO
Copy no. 1	DATE OF ISSUE	DURATION: dd/mm/yyyy to dd/mm/yyyy		Organisation Name

Activity Particulars					Plan of Work (Status: Accomplished = Y; Not-Accomplished = N)												
					MONTH 1								MONTH 2				
Activity	Person Responsible	Signatures	Start Date	End Date	1st week		2nd week		3rd week		4th week		1st week		2nd week		Comments
					Plans	Status	Plans	Status	Plans	Status	Plans	Status	Plans	Status	Plans	Status	
A.1	Mr. X		dd/mm	dd/mm	A.1.1	Y/N	A.1.1 A.1.2	Y/N Y/N	A.1.1 A.1.2	Y/N Y/N	A.1.2	Y/N					
A.2	Ms. Y		dd/mm	dd/mm	A.2.1	Y/N	A.2.1 A.2.2 A.2.3	Y/N Y/N Y/N	A.2.1 A.2.2 A.2.3	Y/N Y/N Y/N	A.2.1 A.2.3	Y/N Y/N	A.2.3	Y/N			
A.3	Mr. Z		dd/mm	dd/mm			A.3.1	Y/N	A.3.2	Y/N	A.3.3	Y/N					
A.4	Ms. A		dd/mm	dd/mm			A.4.1 A.4.2	Y/N	A.4.2 A.4.3	Y/N	A.4.2 A.4.3	Y/N	A.4.2	Y/N			
A.5	Ms. Y		dd/mm	dd/mm									A.5.1 A.5.2	Y/N Y/N	A.5.1	Y/N	
A.6	Mr. X		dd/mm	dd/mm											A.6.1	Y/N	

	Name	Signature	Date
Author	Mr. XXX		
Q.A. Review	Mr. YYY		
Management Approval	**Dr. ZZZ**		

Fig. 6.1 Sample Master Schedule for individual project

MASTER SCHEDULE (Facility) [Screenshot of Half Year's Schedule]			Data Controller (Signature/Stamp)	Organisation LOGO Organisation Name
Copy no. 1	DATE OF ISSUE	Year		

Project Particulars						Plan of Work (Status: Achieved = Y; Not-Achieved = N)												
						Phase of Project *												Comments
						Month 1 (Jan 2020)		Month 2 (Feb 2020)		Month 3 (March 2020)		Month 4 (April 2020)		Month 5 (May 2020)		Month 6 (June 2020)		
Project	Principal Investigator	Funding Agency	Sign.	Start Date	End Date	Phase (P) & Milestone (M)	Status	Phase (P) & Milestone (M)	Status	Phase (P) & Milestone (M)	Status	Phase (P) & Milestone (M)	Status	Phase (P) & Milestone (M)	Status	Phase (P) & Milestone (M)	Status	
Proj.1	Mr. A	N/A		dd/mm	dd/mm	P-2 M.1 P-2 M.2	Y/N Y/N	P-2 M.3 P-2 M.4 P-3 M.1	Y/N Y/N Y/N	P-3 M.2 P-3 M.3	Y/N Y/N	P-4 M.1 P-4 M.2	Y/N Y/N	P-4 M.3 P-5 M.1	Y/N Y/N	P-5 M.2 P-5 M.3	Y/N Y/N	
Proj.2	Ms. B	DST		dd/mm	dd/mm	P-3 M.1 P-3 M.2	Y/N Y/N	P-3 M.3 P-4 M.1	Y/N Y/N	P-4 M.2 P-4 M.3	Y/N Y/N	P-4 M.4 P-4 M.5	Y/N Y/N	P-5 M.1 P-5 M.2 P-5 M.3	Y/N Y/N Y/N			
Proj.3	Mr. C	N/A		dd/mm	dd/mm			P-1 M.1	Y/N	P-1 M.2 P-1 M.3	Y/N Y/N	P-2 M.1 P-2 M.2 P-2 M.3	Y/N Y/N Y/N	P-3 M.1 P-3 M.2 P-3 M.3	Y/N Y/N Y/N	P-3 M.4 P-4 M.1 P-4 M.2	Y/N Y/N Y/N	
Proj.4	Ms. D	ICMR		dd/mm	dd/mm			P-1 M.1 P-1 M.2	Y/N Y/N	P-1 M.3 P-2 M.1	Y/N Y/N	P-2 M.2	Y/N	P-3 M.1 P-3 M.2	Y/N Y/N			
Proj.5	Ms. B	N/A		dd/mm	dd/mm									P-1 M.1 P-1 M.2	Y/N Y/N	P-2 M.1 P-2 M.2 P-2 M.3	Y/N Y/N Y/N	

	Name	Signature	Date
Author	Mr. XXX		
Q.A. Review	Mr. YYY		
Management Approval	**Dr. ZZZ**		

***** Refer "S.O.Ps for Facility Master Schedule & Master Schedule of Individual Project for details on their Phases"*

Fig. 6.2 Sample Master Schedule for the whole facility

Detailed Work Schedule Project: XXXXX			Team Lead / Principle Investigator
Copy no. 1	DATE OF ISSUE	Period of Work dd/mm/yyyy to dd/mm/yyyy	Name: .... Signature: ....

Work Particulars		Plan of Work with Milestones (M)								RESOURCES required with details & date of introduction	Comments
Objective (O) & Activity (A)	Name of Researcher	1st week	2nd week	3rd week	4th week	5th week	6th week	7th week	8th week		
O-1 A.1											
O-1 A.2											
O-1 A.3											
O-1 A.4											
O-1 A.5											
O-2 A.1											
O-2 A.2											
O-2 A.3											
O-3 A.1											
O-3 A.2											
O-3 A.3											
O-3 A.4											
O-3 A.5											
O-3 A.6											
O-4 A.1											
O-4 A.2											
Additional Activities											

	Name	Signature	Date
Author			
Q.A. Review			
Management Approval			

Fig. 6.3 Sample Detailed Work Schedule (DWS)

on the amount of information you want to add to the Master Schedule. The main body of Master Schedule in general contains the following information:

1. **Study name with study Code**
   Title of the study can be mentioned on the master schedule. However, in cases where confidentiality needs to be maintained, a unique identification code is provided to the study and mentioned in the master schedule. The details of such codes are provided to QA.
2. **Date of the study initiation**
   Initiation date of the project is usually the date when the study was signed by the study director and principal investigators (in case of multicentric study). The progress records of the project are maintained effective from this date onward.
3. **Study director**
   Details of the study director assigned for the study including his name, contact, and address should be mentioned. In the case of multicentric study, another column with the name of the principal investigator for the site where the master schedule is generated and managed should be added.
4. **Study Sponsor**
   The master schedule also contains details related to the sponsor for the study such as the name of the agency, contact, and address. In case of a need to maintain confidentiality, a unique identification code specific to the sponsor can be mentioned.
5. **Test system**
   Test system as defined in OECD guidelines is "any biological, chemical or physical system or a combination thereof used in a study" [3]. For example, if the study involves an animal testing system, species and strain of the animals should be mentioned wherever applicable.
6. **Test Article**
   Test article, the substance being tested, and its detail that are felt necessary for project assessment are also included in the master schedule sheet. Example: Drug A given intra-muscular, intravenous, or subcutaneous.
7. **Table containing date and activity**
   Log of all the activities committed in the tabular form (divided weekly or daily as per laboratory and protocol requirement) should be given. It should contain the detail of activity to be performed, initiation date of activity, status (complete or incomplete), and completion date (if applicable). This table will give highlights of all the activities committed for the month and volume of work expected to be completed at the end.
8. **Revision of Master Schedule**
   If the master schedule is a revised version of the earlier master schedule, a review date should be mentioned. An updated copy of master schedule should be provided to QA for his record-keeping and archiving.
9. **Study Director/QA approval**
   The last section of master schedule should include the signature of the study director and management that indicates their approval and responsibility to provide infrastructure and signature of research personnel for his commitment to the work.

Besides these major heads, every laboratory or study can include further information as per their requirement they consider appropriate such as study report issue date and the date of archiving.

6.3 Utility of Master Schedule in Research Productivity

1. **Track of project progress:**
   The main purpose of master schedule is to provide a synopsis of ongoing work and its progress. Monthly commitment at the beginning and evaluation at the end of each month makes it quite easy for QA and the study director to keep a track of project. The estimation of deliverables at end of the month gives a fair idea of how many project milestones are expected to be achieved in a time-bound manner and helps decision-makers to take timely corrective actions in case of delays.
2. **Tool for Quality Assurance inspection:**
   QA personnel invariably use the master schedule as a tool to evaluate the work progress and quality of work during its monthly inspection. Observations about the work progress, taking into consideration the timeline of master schedule for few consecutive months, clearly reflects the irregularities in the project and helps in investigating the reason for such irregularities.
3. **Performance assessment of Research personnel:**
   The performance of research personnel working on the project can be evaluated using the master schedule. The adherence to schedule shows her commitment toward the work. Tasks on her master schedule give highlights of activities she was involved in during that month.
4. **Replanning and better execution of project:**
   Another purpose that master schedule serves is to indicate the need for replanning in ongoing projects. Master schedule in a way reflects the amount of quality work achievable in a month. Complete/incomplete task ratio from the master schedule helps to replan the remaining work in a better way. A much better planning leads to better execution in the following months. During this replanning process, the management gets fair cues about the need for resource reallocation or additions and timely intervention prevents further delays in the project.
5. **Reference for future research projects:**
   Master schedules of all the projects are archived at the end of the project along with all documents related to that project. These then act as a history record that can serve as a reference for the planning and execution of future projects.

Master Schedules are being efficiently utilized by researchers all over the world to ensure enhanced quality of research, be it a simple research project or a complete program encompassing various research projects. There have been numerous innovative ways this important instrument of GLP has been customized and utilized by researchers. Tyagi and Anand while demonstrating their innovative ZED-YOG quality module as a management tool used master schedules to ensure the quality of their research [4]. Crosby puts Master Schedules on the list of most practical and easy-to-use time-management techniques for Physicians in their office and research work [5]. The Neuroscience Research Lab at one of the premier healthcare institutes of India has been awarded by Nation's Quality Council for setting examples for others by implementing the quality principles through practices such as master scheduling and others [6]. Nigg et al. in their work have concluded that a systematic approach that includes formative, evaluation, and summative strategies utilizing tools like master schedule is crucial to the effective development of emerging research centers [7].

6.4 Master Schedule and Research Personnel

GLP requires its research personnel to have competence in the tasks that they are supposed to handle (training and experience). Master schedule can be a valuable instrument to evaluate the performance of the research personnel. Signing a Master schedule means that you understand the task in hand and are responsible for efficient fulfillment of it. Master schedule gives a glimpse of the volume of work done and by which person. Research personnel working on the same project will have a similar project code and the activities performed by each of them will be listed in master schedule reflecting the workload of each personnel. Management can decide on shifting a workload from one to another depending on his evaluation and weightage of load on each individual.

6.5 Master Schedule and Study Director

Once the study has been approved and signed by the study director and management, protocols have been developed, it enters the master scheduling phase. Signing by the study director makes him fully responsible to ensure that the resources (human resource, space, instrumentation, chemicals, etc.) required by personnel are provided to him as per GLP guidelines. Allocation of lab resources is the responsibility of management and therefore in GLP, this resource allocation is documented on the Master Schedule as well.

In a multisite study, the Master schedule should be prepared for each site with the unique study code for the project mentioned at each site. Master schedule will indicate what activities are performed at each site. The study director should be mentioned on all master schedules and the principal investigator responsible for each site on respective master schedules. It is usually the responsibility of the principal investigator of that site to allocate necessary resources for those activities. The master schedule for such projects provides an insight into the workload at each site and helps management in the recruitment of research personnel at each site.

6.6 Master Schedule as a Quality Tool: Recording Deviations in Master Schedule

The master schedule is maintained till the study director submits the final report duly signed to the management and this will be considered as the completion date of the project. Thus, any GLP-related study begins with its entry on master schedule and completes with final report submission as mention on the status of master schedule. Master schedule is therefore a real time tracker for the study in progress. Signed hard copies are usually archived and made available during the inspection by audit committee. QA assessment is based on the adherence or completion of activities listed on the master schedule. Certain headings can be coded instead of directly mentioning them such as sponsor or product name to keep it confidential. Needless to say, decodes for those codes are available to QA at all times for his independence in the GLP system.

It is, therefore, a commendable document that serves as a quality tool in productivity evaluation in GLP studies. The productivity in a given time period of study can be easily evaluated. Productivity is a measure of performance of the study. Productivity change with time provides the study director with valuable data that can be analyzed to understand the reasons for the change in productivity. These factors can be worked upon and replanning of the project can be done in cases whenever required. For this purpose, the deviations from the master schedule should be recorded at specified periods like at the month end. During quality evaluation, QA can also point out the deviations and concerned research personnel can then mention the reasons for the deviations such as unavailability of resources, time or space constraint, postponement of task due to some reason, new task added, etc. This will give information on net productivity in the month.

When more than one research project is being carried out in a test facility, the management registers all the ongoing studies on the master schedule. The master schedule of all the studies carried out in the test facility defines the workload at facility based on which management can draw conclusions that whether they can undertake any new project in the test facility meeting. Any deviation in the individual Master Schedules must be entered into the Facility Master Schedule and further decision making be done based on these. The sufficiency of means required to conduct the extra study at the facility concurrently with the ongoing projects is met as per the GLP norms. If the management decides to enter a new contract, it becomes obliged to provide research staff, room for tests, and chemicals to run the project. Any mismanagement on any part will be considered as a folly of management and, therefore, master schedule provides management with the power to take the best decision (whether to enter a new contract) in their vested interest.

6.7 Tools and Techniques That Go Handy with Master Schedule

There are many management tools and techniques which help management personnel in planning, operations, and evaluation of any project [8–11]. Commonly used scheduling tools include:

- Schedule Network Analysis (Gantt Chart, PERT)
- Critical Path Method (CPM)
- Critical Chain Method (CCM)
- Schedule Compression
- What-if scenario
- Resource leveling

All the timeline tools used in a project invariably have certain key elements which include task (activity), task duration, task dependencies dates related to tasks (start, end, milestones), and task assignees. These are self-explanatory.

Schedule Network Analysis tools like Gantt Chart and PERT help in identifying and representing the feasible timelines set for all the activities to be undertaken for productive research and thus prove to be a great aid in project scheduling. These are graphical representation of all activities of the project, the time allocated to each, and the sequence in which they need to be accomplished besides providing the interrelationships between them. Gantt and PERT are commonly used formats for Schedule Network Analysis and have been depicted in Figs. 6.4 and 6.5. Gantt charts are typically a bar graph of activities depicting the start–end dates, duration of activities, and milestones while PERT is an arrow and node diagram of activities and events; arrows representing the "activities" required to reach each "event," i.e., the nodes which depict each completed phase of the project.

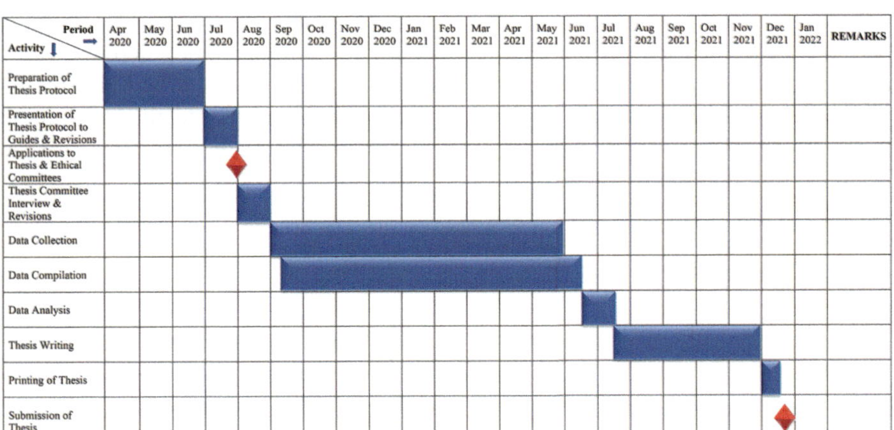

Fig. 6.4 A simple Gant Chart for a thesis research work

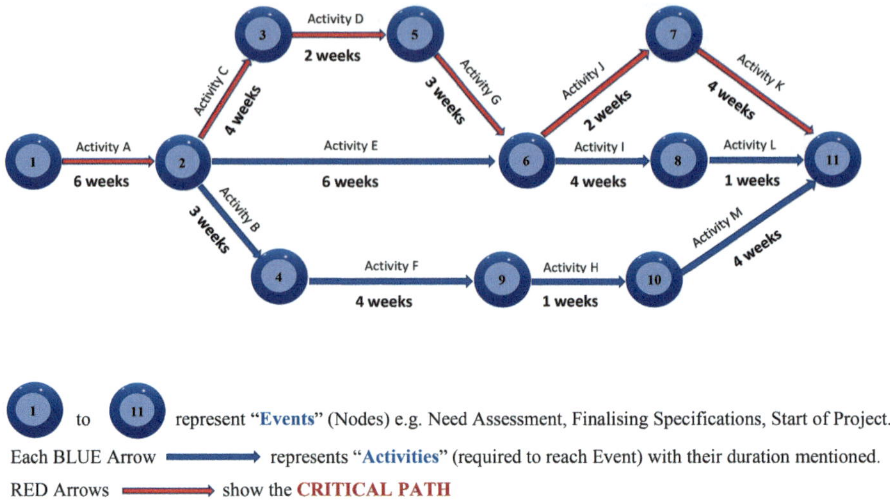

Fig. 6.5 PERT and CPM

CPM and Critical Chain Method elucidate the critical activities (on timeline) on which the overall progress of the project depends the most and any deviation from such identified activities would invariably hamper the productivity [12].CPM provides for the "longest stretch" of dependent activities amongst all the dependent activities (Fig. 6.5). It measures the time (from start to end) required to accomplish this stretch of activities which is "critical" to the progress of the project and any delays in which would cause delayed completion of the project. CPM has been depicted in Fig. 6.5. PERT and CPM are complementary tools and usually used together. Schedule compression tools are used to decrease the time allocated to some of the activities thereby reducing the total duration of the project.

These tools should be used to supplement any Master Schedule. These are established tools for efficient management for ages. And when utilized in tune with the master schedule, can ensure a high level of efficiency in research productivity. There are numerous software and online tools available to assist researchers in developing and utilizing these techniques in their projects. Discussing the details about these tools is beyond the scope of this chapter and interested readers may refer to the available literature on the same.

6.8 Technology and Master Scheduling

As we have already discussed, a number of software and online tools are readily available today for the researchers to efficiently utilize the project time-management tools for enhanced research productivity. Technology has made master scheduling very easy and effective. Some examples of project management timeline software that can be used for devising efficient Master Schedules include Nifty, nTasks,

Psoda, Quire, GanttPro, Smartsheet, Wrike, Bitrix24, ProofHub, Workzone, EasyProjects, Celoxis, Office Timeline, etc.

Besides this, there are many applications (Apps) available to assist researchers in developing and keeping a real-time track of the Master Schedules. Commonly used ones include Asana, Trello, OmniPlan, Casual, Basecamp, Podio, Microsoft Project, etc.

Depending upon ease of use, suitability, features, and charges, one may choose amongst the many available software/apps to assist in developing and executing Master Schedules. They help in real-time management through Master Schedules and enhance research productivity of individual/organization by assisting in task management, time tracking, issues management, risk management, resource planning and management, feedback management, reporting, performance evaluation and prioritizing. Additional features like data export, interactive interface, risk analytics, project budgeting, email invites, multi-lingulate, notes, search functionality, role-based permissions, customizable templates automatic notifications, computer telephony, meeting scheduling and management, etc. are proving to be a boon to the research fraternity today. Most of the available software and tools come along with a training program to provide hassle-free hands-on on its use to the researcher.

6.9 Future Direction and Implications

Researchers worldwide face a challenge of global acceptance of the data generated at their end as good quality of research has been a crucial prerequisite for becoming acceptable to the scientists. Principles of Good laboratory practices of OECD are internationally accepted norms [13] for quality research that makes your data widely recognition. Master Schedule is one important module of the Good Lab practices (GLP) which can considerably help the researchers to maintain the quality of data. It empowers the researcher by keeping a track record of the progress of the project and therefore enhanced efficiency in the work. Information reflected from the Master Schedule of a project aids the quality assurance person to note any discrepancy in the work and ensures that corrective actions are taken well in time. Grand Master Schedule containing information from all the projects undergoing in the research facility gives an idea about the total workload at the test facility and also helps the inspection committee to assess the quality and management to take a valuable decision regarding expansion or retrenchment of work. Master Schedule is, therefore, a tool that is handy for quality control at all levels of hierarchy whether it is research personnel, quality assurance personnel, or management. Archived Master schedule records when matched with other GLP modules like SOP and DRS make the data generated at the test facility at a given timepoint verifiable at each step and add more weightage to it. Rigid GLP norms exploiting managerial tools such as Master schedule will make researchers more confident in the presentation of their data and more acceptable to the advanced groups involved in research. Pharmaceutical companies would be more appreciative of such data being produced in GLP regulated manner and in turn boost their confidence in investing in clinical trials based on results coming from such studies.

References

1. World Health Organization. Handbook: good laboratory practice (GLP): quality practices for regulated non-clinical research and development. World Health Organization; 2010.
2. Carson PA, Dent NJ, editors. Good clinical, laboratory and manufacturing practices: techniques for the QA professional. Cambridge: Royal Society of Chemistry; 2007.
3. Goeke J. The master schedule index. In: Good clinical, laboratory and manufacturing practices. Cambridge: Royal Society of Chemistry; 2017. p. 199–207.
4. Tyagi R, Anand A. Development and implementation of ZED-YOG quality module: Niyantrita Madhumeha Bharata skill development initiatives. Ann Neurosci. 2019;26(1):37–44.
5. Crosby JW. Ten time-management tips for family physicians. CMAJ Can Med Assoc J. 2004;170(6):949–50.
6. Anand A. National model for replicating benchmarking of basic research investigations in govt institutes: a case for ministries of science and technology and health and family welfare. Ann Neurosci. 2014;21(2):41.
7. Nigg CR, Qureshi K, Inouye J, Sy A, Sullivan K, Boland MG. Evaluation of an emerging research center: lessons learned. Int J Res Nurs. 2012;3(1):1–7.
8. APM. Association for Project Management body of knowledge. 6th ed. High Wycombe, UK: Association for Project Management; 2012.
9. IPMA. ICB-IPMA competence baseline version 3.0. Nijkerk, The Netherlands: International Project Management Association (IPMA); 2006.
10. PMI. A guide to the project management body of knowledge. 5th ed. P. M. I. N. square. USA, ed. Newtown Square, PA: Project Management Institute; 2008.
11. Herroelen W, Leus R. On the merits and pitfalls of critical chain scheduling. J Oper Manag. 2001;19(5):559–77.
12. Kumar A, Chakraborty BS. Application of critical path analysis in clinical trials. J Adv Pharm Technol Res. 2016;7(1):17–21.
13. Seiler JP. Good laboratory practice: the why and the how. Berlin: Springer; 2006.

7 Logsheets and the Academic Progress of Ph.D. Students

Kalyan Maity and K. Sadasivan Pillai

7.1 Introduction

The irreproducibility of research is a severe crisis that the research community is facing today. A survey conducted on 1576 researchers revealed that more than 70% of them failed to reproduce another researcher's experiments, and more than half have failed to reproduce their own experiments [1, 2]. The reasons attributed to the irreproducibility of research are many. One of the reasons is improper or no recording of experimental details. An experiment may fail due to the use of expired reagents, non-calibrated equipment, non-validated methods, poor experimental conditions, etc. If the researcher wants to investigate the failure or reassure the success of the experiment, he/she should have evidence of the conduct of all the activities related to the experiment, which include the reagents and equipment used, environmental conditions maintained while conducting the experiment, etc. For the conduct of any experiment, it is essential to maintain traceable records of the thought process of the experimenter and the detailed procedures of the experiments [3]. The experimenter should ensure that such records made are accurate, complete, and accessible.

In a research laboratory adhering to the principles of GLP (Good Laboratory Practice), recording of these activities is done in logsheets. Logsheet is defined as

K. Maity
Division of Yoga and Life Sciences, Swami Vivekananda Yoga Anusandhana Samsthana (S-VYASA), Bengaluru, Karnataka, India

Neuroscience Research Laboratory, Department of Neurology, PGIMER, Chandigarh, Chandigarh, India

K. S. Pillai (✉)
Scientific Advisory Board, International Institute of Biotechnology and Toxicology, Padappai, Tamil Nadu, India
e-mail: pillaiksp@yahoo.com

A. Anand (ed.), *Quality Assurance Implementation in Research Labs*,
https://doi.org/10.1007/978-981-16-3074-3_7

the data recording tool to record each and every information of any particular activity. The entry of activity in a logsheet should be made as and when it occurs. Logsheets provide confidence to the experimenter about the work/activity that he/she had carried out. Logsheets are proof of the past activity performed. For easy maintenance, a separate logsheet is maintained for each activity.

7.2 Laboratory Notebook and Logsheet

It is a usual practice in several academic institutions to record experimental procedures and findings in a laboratory notebook [4]. A Laboratory notebook (LNB) is a controlled document; hence, the experimenter should get it issued from his/her mentor or document controller. The pages of the LNB are numbered, and a separate space is allotted to write the title of the experiment, aim and objectives of the experiment, instruments and materials to be used for the conduct of the experiment, results, interpretation/conclusion, and dated signature of the experimenter. Each experiment is given a title and unique number in the LNB, which is useful in recording an activity related to the experiment in logsheets. Several industrial research laboratories have implemented a paperless recording system, by establishing electronic laboratory notebooks [5]. But electronic laboratory notebook has some risk in maintaining intellectual properties [6]. A major difficulty in implementing an electronic laboratory notebook is that all laboratory equipment are required to be software based in order to communicate with each other. In today's quality system, it is a requirement that all software is validated, which is an expensive and difficult task for an academic research laboratory.

LNB provides elaborate details of experiments done, whereas logsheet provides evidence of various activities of the experiments performed. Therefore, a well-designed scientific experiment explained in an LNB loses its scientific credential, if the records of the activities of the experiment done are not traceable.

Broadly the logsheets maintained in academic research laboratories can be classified into personal logsheets and laboratory logsheets. In this chapter, a brief description of the logsheets maintained in academic research laboratories is given. Templates of a few of the logsheets maintained in our laboratory (Neuroscience Research Laboratory, Department of Neurology, PGIMER, Chandigarh-160012, India) are also presented in the chapter.

7.3 Personal Logsheets

7.3.1 Journal Clubs Attended/Journal Clubs Presented

Presenting published research papers of other authors related to the Ph.D. student's research area at the journal club is an important part of research activity. While presenting the paper, it is expected that the research student discusses what is

Table 7.1 Journal club attended/journal club presented—logsheet template

Name	Date of Joining	Position Held	Venue	Date and Time
*Journal Club Attended/Presented	Name of the Speaker		Title of the Topic	
Key Points Discussed (use a separate sheet if necessary):				
Signature of the Attendee		Signature of the Speaker		
Format No		*Format Approving Date*		

***Strike off as appropriate**

lacking in that study and what could further be done in that study. While studying and presenting another researcher's work, one can improve his/her style of presentation of research findings. Another benefit is that the research student can improve his/her presentation skills, both in writing scientific articles and giving oral presentations. By attending and taking part in discussions in the journal club, the research student learns to formulate questions to be asked in scientific platforms. The research student should keep a record of the journal club attended and the presentation made in the journal in the logsheet. The record should detail the speaker's name, the title of the topic of the research paper presented, the date of the presentation, and the venue where the Journal club was held. It is also important to mention in the logsheet the key points discussed in the journal club (Table 7.1).

7.3.2 Seminars Attended/Seminars Presented

In the seminar, the student should present research papers, usually related to his/her research work, and discuss the research findings. The presentation of negative results obtained from the experiments should be encouraged in the seminars. The research student may cite other scientists' work to support his/her findings, but it is expected that the student also explains the findings using his/her thought process.

As for the Journal club mentioned above, a similar record of seminars attended and seminars presented should be maintained in the logsheet.

7.3.3 Research Meetings Attended

Attending research meetings helps to solve the problems that regress research progress and encountered in other related activities. The research meeting logsheet provides information on the discussion held in the meeting and also provides an indication of the agenda to be discussed in the next meeting. A template of logsheet for the research meeting attended is given in Table 7.2.

7.3.4 Laboratory Meetings Attended

In the laboratory meetings, research students have a discussion with the PI about any issue in the laboratory, and the progress made in the research work till the date. Logsheets of such meetings should be maintained (Table 7.3).

Table 7.2 Research meeting attended—logsheet template

Name	Date of Joining	Position Held	Venue	Date and Time
Key Points Discussed (use a separate sheet if necessary):				
Signature of the Attendee		Signature of the Supervisor/Mentor		
Format No		*Format Approving Date*		

Table 7.3 Laboratory meeting attended—logsheet template

Name of the Student	Date of Joining	Position Held	Venue	Date and Time
Title of the Research Topic				
Key Points Discussed (use a separate sheet if necessary):				
Signature of the Student		Signature of the Supervisor/Mentor		
Format No		*Format Approving Date*		

7.3.5 Research Data Presented

The raw data should be presented in an effective format. It can be presented in textual, tabular, or graphical forms, depending on the nature of the data. It is very important to select an appropriate method to present raw data [7]. Ph.D. students should consider several rules while presenting the raw data, especially numerical data, for example, the number of figures to be retained after the decimal point. It is also important to present results of statistical analysis with proper justification, for example, standard error and standard deviation, significant level denoted as $P < 0.05$, etc. A separate logsheet should be established for making entries of details of such meetings (Table 7.4).

7.3.6 Leave Records

Planned leave should be recorded in the logsheet and all concerned should be informed so that the ongoing work does not get affected. Any unplanned leave should be informed to a colleague, who will take care of the research activity of the leave applicant in his/her absence, if required; both are required to put signatures in the leave application logsheet (Table 7.5).

Table 7.4 Research data presented—logsheet template

Name of the Student	Date of Joining	Position Held	Venue	Date and Time
Title of the Research Topic			*Raw Data Format	Textual Tabular Graphical Statistical Analysis
Raw Data Description (Example, Bodyweight, IgG, Statistical analysis, etc.)				
Key Points Discussed (use a separate sheet if necessary):				
Signature of the Student		Signature of the Supervisor/Mentor		
Format No		*Format Approving Date*		

*Put a tick mark in the appropriate box given in the next column

7.3.7 Details of Work Done on Different Projects

In case a research student is working on a project other than his/her research work, it should be documented in the logsheet. This information is useful in assessing the workload of the research student. Assessing such workload is necessary to maintain the quality of the research activities in the department, because quality may be compromised in the work of a student overburdened with several projects. A template of the logsheet for recording details of the work done and time utilized for other projects is provided in Table 7.6.

Table 7.5 Leave application—logsheet template

Name of the Student			Date of Joining	Position Held	
Date of Leave Required (Panned Leave) or Absence (Unplanned Leave)[1]	Leave Type-Planned (P) or Unplanned (UP)	Reason for the Leave	Signature of the Personnel[2]	Signature of the Leave Applicant	Signature of the Approving Authority
Format No			*Format Approving Date*		

[1]Fill in the date of unplanned leave on joining the lab work after the leave
[2]The person who performed the work in the absence of the leave applicant

Table 7.6 Work done and time utilized in other projects—logsheet template

Name of the Student			Date of Joining	Position Held		
Date	Title of the Project	Details of the Work Done		Time Utilized for the Work (h)	Signature of the Student	Signature of the Supervisor/ Mentor
Format No			*Format Approving Date*			

Table 7.7 Doctoral committee meetings—logsheet template

Name of the Student	Date of Joining	Position Held	Venue	Date and Time
Title of the Research Topic				
Key Points Discussed (use a separate sheet if necessary):				
Signature of the Student		Signature of the Supervisor/Mentor		
Format No		*Format Approving Date*		

Table 7.8 Research paper communicated/published—logsheet template

Name of the Student			Date of Joining	Position Held				
Serial Number	Title of the Paper	Authors	Journal Name	Publication Status[1]			Date Copy of the Paper Submitted to Dept Library[2]	Signature of the Student
				Communicate	Under	Published		
Format No			*Format Approving Date*					

[1]Put a tick mark in the appropriate subcolumn
[2]Write NA (Not applicable), if the paper is not published

7.3.8 Doctoral Committee Meetings

A separate logsheet should be maintained to record the presentations made or the discussion held at the Doctoral committee meetings (Table 7.7).

Table 7.9 Conferences participated—logsheet template

Name of the Student	Date of Joining	Position Held	Address of Conference Venue	Date and Time
Name of the Conference				
Research Paper Presented[1]	Oral	Poster	Participated as an Observer	
Title of Research Paper Presented				
Key Take away messages from the conference (use a separate sheet if necessary):				
Signature of the Student		Signature of the Supervisor/Mentor		
Format No		*Format Approving Date*		

[1]Put a tick mark in the appropriate box given in the next column

7.3.9 Research Papers Communicated/Published

A record of research papers communicated/published should be maintained in a logsheet (Table 7.8).

7.3.10 Conferences Participated

A record of participation in conferences should be maintained in a logsheet (Table 7.9).

7.3.11 Meetings Held with Visiting/Guest Faculties

Another way to expand one's knowledge is by meeting and discussing with guest faculties. The research student should formulate the questions to be asked or doubts to be cleared with the guest faculty in advance. Such meetings should be captured in the logsheet. The template of the logsheet for meeting with visiting/guest faculties is similar to that given in Table 7.7.

7.3.12 Discussion with PI

Record in the logsheet the periodic discussions held with the PI. The problems faced in experimental work and difficulty in understanding scientific aspects in the research subject should be discussed with the PI. List out all the matters to be discussed with the PI prior to the meeting. The template of the logsheet for holding discussions with PI is similar to that given in Table 7.7.

7.3.13 Community Services

All research work should ultimately benefit society, mankind, or the environment. Any work carried out in this direction should be captured in a logsheet.

7.4 Laboratory Logsheets

7.4.1 Equipment Maintenance and Operation

In the quality system of a research laboratory, the equipment logsheet occupies a prominent position as it provides history, day-to-day performance including breakdown, maintenance, calibration, and validation status of the equipment. Equipment logsheet is the only means by which the researcher can assure the reliability and

Table 7.10 Equipment maintenance and operation—logsheet template

Equipment Name		**Manufacturer**		**Serial Number**		**Date of Purchase.**		**Equipment SOP No.**	
Equipment User Manual No.		**Validation Date and Validation Document Location (Folder No.)**		**Revali dation Date**		**External Calibration Documents Location (Folder No.)**		**Equipment Location**	
Date	User Name		Purpose	Login Time		Logout Time	Remarks[a]		User Signature
Format No						*Format Approving Date*			

[a]A tick mark in Remarks column indicates the Equipment was working satisfactorily at the time of logout

accuracy of the data obtained from the equipment. A template of the equipment logsheet is given in Table 7.10.

An equipment logsheet should contain equipment-related details like the name, manufacturer, and serial number of the equipment. It is useful to mention the date of purchase of the equipment as it provides an indication of the age of the equipment. The due date for calibration may be decided based on the age and frequency of use of the equipment. The equipment manual is a document as important as the SOP of the equipment. The IQ/OQ/PQ of the equipment must also be noted at the time of purchase of equipment. In a GLP research laboratory, the equipment manual is given a unique identification number and treated as a controlled document. Mention in the logsheet where the equipment is located. Small pieces of equipment like pipettes, hygrometers, thermometers, etc., can be shifted from one place to the other, but equipment of higher levels including weighing balances should not be shifted often from one place to the other. If there is a need for shifting, calibrate the equipment before use. Mention in the logsheet where the validation and external calibration documents are stored. The day-to-day activities are recorded promptly in the appropriate columns: in the column titled "Purpose," experiment number, project number, calibration, preventive maintenance, repairs, etc., are entered as the case may be. In the column titled "Remarks," a tick mark is added if the equipment is working satisfactorily, otherwise the problem encountered with the equipment is described.

Table 7.11 Animal house activities—logsheet template

Observations Made/ Activities Carried Out	Date and Time																														
Recording of Room temp.& Humidity																															
Floor cleaning																															
Physical Examination																															
Bed change																															
Cage change																															
Drinking water bottle change																															
Feeding																															
Watering																															
Mortality observed/ Carcass removed																															
Sacrifice																															
Signature																															
Format No													*Format Approving Date*																		

√ Observation made/Activity done; × Observation not made/Activity not done

7.4.2 Laboratory Environmental Monitoring

Biological samples are sensitive to a change in environmental conditions in the laboratory. The environmental conditions, particularly temperature and humidity should be set to the accepted range so that sample handling, analysis, and equipment operation are not affected by the change in temperature and humidity. Controlling environmental conditions in animal house facilities is essential as a small change in the environmental condition may adversely affect the outcome of the study [8, 9]. The temperature and humidity of the analytical laboratory and animal house should be recorded in the logsheet. Evaluation of microbial contamination is necessary for the laboratories handling biological materials and in the animal house facilities. All the activities done in the animal house should be reflected in a logsheet (Table 7.11).

7.4.3 Microbiology Media/Reagent

Details of the chemicals or reagents prepared should be captured in logsheets. In the case of preparation of media, record at least the following in the logsheet [10]:

- Date and preparer's name
- Expiry date
- Storage condition
- Name of the medium, the lot number, and manufacturer
- Number of prepared plates, tubes, bottles, or flasks
- Assigned lot and batch numbers
- Color, consistency, and appearance
- Number of plates used for QC
- Sterility test results at 24 and 48 h
- Growth test(s)
- pH
- In the case of preparation of a reagent, record the following in the logsheet:
- Date and preparer's name
- Expiry date
- Storage condition
- Assigned number
- Color and appearance (if applicable)

Table 7.12 Chemical inventory—logsheet template

Location:		**Month:**		
Maintained by:		**Updated on:**		
Sr. No.	Name of Chemical	**Company**	**Quantity**	**Number**
1.				
2.				
Personnel Involved	**Name**		**Signature**	
Prepared by				
Reviewed by				
Reviewed by QA				
Format No.		*Format Approving Date*		

Table 7.13 Sample (test item) storage, issuance, and disposal—logsheet template

Sample (Test Item) Collected/ Received by	Date of Collection	Quantity of Sample Received (provide units)	Describe Container in Which Sample Received	Storage Condition (Freeze, Refrigerate, Room Temperature)	Stored in (Identification No. of Freezer, Refrigerator, Cupboard etc)	Sample (TI) Disposal (Describe quantity of TI disposed, Method of disposal, Reason for disposal with signature)
Date	Issued to	Quantity Issued (provide units)	Opening Stock (provide units)	Balance Stock (provide units)	Signature	
Format No.				*Format Approving Date*		

7.4.4 Chemical Inventory

Logsheet is an essential tool for judicious use and for maintaining an inventory of high purity chemicals. The entries in the logsheet should be made in such a way that at any time point the information on the quantity of the chemicals is readily available (Table 7.12).

7.4.5 Sample (Test Item) and Reference Items

A sample is the key substance of the research; hence, it should be collected, transported, stored, prepared (formulated), and disposed of appropriately. Records of all

Table 7.14 Materials disposal—logsheet template

Serial No.	Date	Material[1]	Quantity[2]	Disposal Method[3]	Source[4]	Signature[5]
Format no.			*Format approving date*			

[1]Mention name of the material to be disposed (e.g., carcass of rats, microbiological nutrient media, animal house bedding material etc.)
[2]Mention quantity of material to be disposed
[3]If an inhouse method is used, mention SOP number. If handed over to an agency approved by the Pollution Control Board, mention so
[4]Mention experiment or project number, if the material is originated from it. If an expired material cannot be traced to an experiment or project, mention as 'expired' with expiry date
[5]The person who puts the signature must ensure that the disposal is done properly

these activities should be available in the logsheet. A template of logsheet for sample (Test Item) is given in Table 7.13.

7.4.6 Coding

Coding of the experiment or test item plays an important role in maintaining the confidentiality and avoiding bias in the research. Any coding activity done should be recorded in a logsheet.

7.4.7 Data Collection

Mistakes in data entry can be avoided by the use of a logsheet [11]. The data varies from one type of experiment to the other. Hence, a structured template may not suit every experiment [4]. In such cases, provisions should be given in the templates to record all types of data.

Table 7.15 Document change control—logsheet template

Change Control Serial Number		
Date		
Document Type (SOP, Format, Study Plan, Others-Specify)		
Document Number		
Title of the Document		
Change/s Proposed	**Existing Procedure**	**Reason for the Change/s**
Initiated by (Name and Signature)	**Laboratory Incharge (Name and Signature)**	**Reviewed by QA (Name and Signature)**
Format no.		*Format approving date*

7.4.8 Disposal

In a research laboratory, a variety of materials are disposed. Dead animals, microbiological nutrient media, biological wastes, used chemicals are a few of the materials regularly disposed of from a biological research facility. Storage and disposal of the materials should be done in a manner that is safe to the handler and the environment. The appropriate procedures should be in place to ensure that all disposal activities are done in an environment-friendly manner. Records of the materials disposed of should be maintained in a logsheet (Table 7.14).

7.4.9 Change Control of Approved Documents

A provision should be available to make changes in any approved document. This will provide a mechanism for continuous improvement in the procedure described in the document. Any change made in the approved document should be justified, reviewed, approved, and then implemented. The procedure to be followed to make a change in an approved document should be adopted for logsheet as well (Table 7.15).

7.5 Future Directions and Clinical Implications

Irreproducibility of research has become a serious concern for scientific communities, funding agencies, and regulatory bodies. The scenario is the worst in preclinical drug research. Several studies reported that a major reason for the failure of drugs in clinical research is the irreproducibility of preclinical research. It is important to establish a system in research facilities to trace every activity of research. The usual practice is to record the activities in logsheets. Another alternative to this is to record electronically, and any change to electronically recorded entry should be traceable without obscuring the original entry.

7.6 Conclusion

Improper or no recording of activities involved in research is one of the reasons for the irreproducibility. Recording an activity carried out in a logsheet provides evidence of that activity carried out. In today's quality systems, including GLP, it is essential to record all activities in the logsheet, so that the logsheets stand as the evidence for the activities carried out, and also act as a tool for tracking the activities.

Acknowledgments The authors are grateful to Dr. M Baskar, Quality Assurance Department, International Institute of Biotechnology and Toxicology for suggestions and for providing notes on the maintenance of logsheets in GLP-certified facilities.

References

1. Baker M. 1,500 scientists lift the lid on reproducibility. Nature. 2016;533(7604):452–4.
2. Baker M. Reproducibility crisis. Nature. 2016;533(26):353–66.
3. Eisenberg A. Keeping a laboratory notebook. J Chem Educ. 1982;59(12):1045.
4. Willoughby C, Logothetis TA, Frey JG. Effects of using structured templates for recalling chemistry experiments. J Cheminformatics. 2016;8(1):9.
5. Bird CL, Willoughby C, Frey JG. Laboratory notebooks in the digital era: the role of ELNs in record keeping for chemistry and other sciences. Chem Soc Rev. 2013;42(20):8157–75.
6. Ramaseshan S. The computer as a laboratory notebook. Curr Sci. 1996;70(11):950.
7. In J, Lee S. Statistical data presentation. Korean J Anesthesiol. 2017;70(3):267.
8. Guide for the Care and Use of Laboratory Animals. Institute for Laboratory Animal Research. National Research Council, Washington, DC, USA, 1996. https://www.ncbi.nlm.nih.gov/books/NBK232589/
9. Clark JD, Gebhart GF, Gonder JC, Keeling ME, Kohn DF. The 1996 guide for the care and use of laboratory animals. ILAR J. 1997;38(1):41–8.
10. WHO. Laboratory Quality Management System: Handbook. World Health Organization; 2011. https://www.who.int/ihr/publications/lqms_en.pdf
11. Hargie O, Tourish D. Data collection log-sheet methods. Auditing organizational communication: a handbook of research, theory and practice. London: Routledge; 2009.

Instigation and Adherence to the Quality Assurance Program to Avoid Academic Conflicts

8

Priya Battu, Bhavya Mody, Sumit Rana, and Kaushal Sharma

8.1 Introduction: Quality Assurance in Academics

The terms Quality, Quality control, and Quality assurance have different connotations. Quality refers to the degree of excellence of a product or process. Quality control is a process involving the fulfillment of quality standards [1] and quality assurance refers to the maintenance of the quality of any product or service by paying attention to every stage of the process. There are many instances in history where failure to comply with quality led to disastrous mishappenings. One such incident is the grounding of Boeing 737 MAX airliners after around 350 people died in two crashes. There was technical insufficiency and lack of transparency which led to the grounding of the airliner, which was the longest ban on any airliner in the history of aviation [2]. Another incident was the Brumadinho Dam disaster, which resulted in the death of nearly 300 people and many were reported to be missing. The dam was owned by Vale SA and the company knew that the sensors that were installed for keeping a check on the structural integrity of the dam had some problems. But the failure to act upon it led to the catastrophe which claimed the lives of hundreds of people. California wildfires were also caused due to poor quality and aged equipment used by the company which led to the loss of lives and property as

P. Battu · S. Rana
Neuroscience Research Lab, Department of Neurology, Post Graduate Institute of Medical Education and Research, Chandigarh, India

B. Mody
Kasturba Medical College, Manipal Academy of Higher Education, Manipal, Karnataka, India

K. Sharma (✉)
Allergy and Immunology Unit, Advanced Pediatrics Centre, Department of Pediatrics, Post Graduate Institute of Medical Education and Research, Chandigarh, India
e-mail: kksukv@gmail.com

A. Anand (ed.), *Quality Assurance Implementation in Research Labs*,
https://doi.org/10.1007/978-981-16-3074-3_8

well. This also brought liability claims against the company [3]. Sometimes the reputation of corporate and researchers is also marred with such controversies due to jealousy-driven accusations [4, 5], and also falsely claiming the data where lack of proper documentation enhances such allegations. These are examples that show the importance of a quality assurance (QA) program in general to promote the transparency and implementation of adequate QA in the respective domains [6]. QA in academics is also required to prevent the conflicts generated during the process of data generation, filing of grants/projects, and presentation of data in the form of publications and patents [6, 7]. The academic conflicts may range from the inception of research questions in form of the academic project till the outcome of the project including an adopted methodology and processes. There have been many strategies and norms laid down from time to time, at the institutional (conflict among research staff and faculties), national (for the public interest, industrial and governmental benefit), and at the global levels (for International collaboration and commercial benefits) which prevent these conflicts. All these come under the aegis of GLP (Good Lab practices). GLP can help in neutralizing and streamlining the various aspects of research and clinical setup during the complete research tenure where various academic conflicts can arise. Some of the basic protocols must be adopted in research labs to manage the research activities at micro/macro levels by preparing the MS (Master schedules), pertaining SOPs (Standard Operating Protocols), DRSs (Data Recording Sheets), *etc.* where the basic method is provided in a structured format. These are required to maintain the documentation of the process/methodology conducted during the experimentations and also to report deviation(s) from SOPs, if any. Similarly, the copyright of a research idea can avoid initial conflict among National and International collaborators, and can motivate the researchers by expanding the implementation of the idea at the societal and commercial level. Hence, an idea must be secured from false claiming of ownership. Simultaneously, applying for grants/funding based on the research idea and its inferences including both at societal and commercial levels must also be streamline to avoid any probable conflicts by enhancing the transparency of the claim and ensuring its credibility [5]. In this case also, copyrights of an idea can further prevent any conflict among the research group's claim. Data generation, which involves comprehensive experimentations, is also a potential source of conflict among research groups (due to adopted methods and processes used). This can also involve data fraud and false claiming of generated data and/or generation of a novel method, which is not reliable or has been copied. To prevent this, preparing an MS and documentation in DRS during the experimental work (along with any deviation from SOP done or observed) of the project can act as a source of record (with time) and it can help in streamlining the activities that are to be performed in the near future [8]. Hence, Master Schedule (MS) should be formulated carefully under the supervision of the Principal Investigator. However, a Grandmaster schedule (GMS) needs to be followed in case of National and International collaborations to further avoid any conflict at any point of time in the project. SOPs are documents that should be followed while performing research to avoid any deviation and to increase the reproducibility of research. However, reporting and documentation of any deviation while performing an experiment as per SOP are equally important in academics. Data Recording Sheets (DRS) can also aid in record keeping and act as proof of the experiments performed which can be matched with logbook entries of used instruments and chemical logsheets to improve the back traceability of the same. Recording the steps of a procedure while performing experiments is another strategy that can be followed to avoid conflicts in the near future. This not only acts as proof of the experiments being performed but also assures that procedures being followed are correct. Once raw data is generated, it should be entered correctly in the form of electronic files and should be validated timely to assess if there are any variability and wrong entries in the recorded data. Moreover, conflicts can be raised in the presentation of data *i.e.* in the form of publications and Patents among collaborators (both National and International) and the parent Institute. Such documentation can serve as a foundation for the formulation of guidelines. Publication agreement document should contain the particulars and contribution of each author and all the authors must duly sign it. Similarly, for patents, the inventorship form should be procured from the inventors. Hence, GLP is an essential and integrative part of the quality assurance program in the research/academic fraternity that must be followed diligently to avoid any kind of associated conflicts. This chapter attempts to discuss the crucial points in research and associated clinical domains to avoid the tampering of data and false claims, if any. To achieve a better outcome, such norms and guidelines, one needs to impose or follow the well-established (universal and/or institutional) guidelines stringently, without any failure.

8.2 Implementation of QA in Academics

Quality assurance is important in academics because it strengthens the defensive party, in case there are false accusations inspired by negative competition. When grants are filed, only a few are accepted and others are rejected, which might be due to lack of merit, bias and funding agency might doubt the procedure followed. A grant should be extensively reviewed, preferably by adopting the double-blinded reviewing process. Neither the applicant must know the reviewers, nor should the identity of the applicant be revealed at any stage till the declaration of result. An online tracking system may be helpful where reviewers can submit their comments in a timely fashion and the applicant can address them as per the expertise of the PI and the co-PIs mentioned in the project. This can be done to improve the grant application by avoiding any biasness during the evaluation of the grant application at any stage. Similarly, an ethical committee consists of experts from wide areas of discipline who can also provide further insight about ethical aspects in the project, which can enhance the outcome and reproducibility with minimum and appropriate use of methods. An ethical committee review must also be transparent and unbiased and should be done without any delay, so that the project outcome can be delivered on time and the career of a associated Ph.D. student is not affected. The ethical committee should be registered to the national body and should be guided for CTRI registration (Clinical Trials Registry of India) and the date of start of the study. It should monitor the research activity on time to observe compliance, as usually after getting the approval, the researchers do not comply with the ethics. Multiple ethical committees within an institute (without Institutional Review Board, IRB) should be discouraged. Conflicts regarding the rationale of the study should be clearly addressed by the applicants. A clear indication of rejection should be mentioned, and further evaluation of amendments should be considered without much delay so that the grant application can be filed timely (to preserve the research question). Conflicts are also generated due to favoritism during recruitment for various positions, promotions, Ph.D. positions, postdocs, *etc*. Hence, the authorities should outline and follow a transparent procedure for recruitment. Each Institute or university may have different criteria which should be notified to the candidates when inviting them. The criteria should be complied to, and any deviation should be mentioned while declaring the results. Hence, a quality assurance program in such academic processes, implemented by internal and external reviewing mechanisms can enhance the auditability, and prevent any false allegations. Additionally, publication of such reports (done by extensive QA review) in Institutional bulletins can also be published which could be appreciable step toward increasing the transparency and creditability of the processes. Similarly, for awards, a certain criteria need to be in place that should be followed and should not be affected by personal relations. These criteria should be based on the common good of the public, for example, on the basis of how the inventions or discoveries were done by the awardee and translation implication of the discoveries. Awards should be based on the applicability of the discovery rather than the number of publications or citations. Sometimes, the number of citations increases by self-citing a publication or citation by peers or collaborators [9–13]. Hence, the implementation of the QA program to avoid the common practice of false awarding based on self-citation, without justification, can also be done for the overall streamlining of the process of award scrutiny [14, 15]. Sometimes self-citation is also being used to self-propagate the research idea of a group among the scientific fraternity. However, QA could (both internal and external review) play important role in the evaluation of self-citation of research paper/idea, could also enhance the research outcome of the respective research group.

Business-related academic conflicts are also generated during lab testing like routine testing, genetic testing, etc. when the results may vary. Hence, it is better to run the samples in duplicates and validate the results by a third person. Equipment used for testing should be well calibrated, and reagents and chemicals should be of quality standard. Currently, India is running trials for five COVID-19 vaccine candidates. However, the lack of transparency in conducting and regulating such trials brings them under scrutiny. Usually, the information regarding such trials is updated on the Clinical Trials Registry of India (CTRI) . The Covishield vaccine testing by one of the institutes in India seemed to not provide complete information regarding the trials. It also seemed that the institute focused on the safety of the vaccine, rather than efficacy, as is expected from Phase 2 and 3 trials. It is not necessary to share testing protocols, but it surely increases public trust, and such steps are being taken by various companies for COVID-19 vaccines. CTRI details are often not updated and are incomplete. Evaluation of the safety and adverse events associated with such trials is also required. Some scientists believe that information regarding the experts who review such proposals and give recommendations should also be made public. Hence, more transparent data sharing policies are encouraged [16].

Implementation of QA in Clinical Settings

Conflicts are also generated during clinical evaluation of the patient, diagnosis of a disease, and in healthcare settings. Misdiagnosis of a disease can cause a life-threatening situation in addition to causing wastage of resources and money. Taking a second opinion can prevent this. A series of clinical investigations needs to be followed by people with internal and external expertise in the field before concluding with a consensus opinion, to strengthen the diagnostic efficacy. For laboratory diagnosis, internal and external quality assessments can be done. Internal quality control refers to the procedures that compare the results produced within the same laboratory at different times/by different people [17]. External quality assessment refers to the comparison of results with external laboratories (to a peer lab or a reference lab) [18]. Using Quality assessments, the aspects that need to be improved in diagnostic methods can be found out. For example, a study conducted to determine the prevalence and causes of misdiagnosis of tuberculosis by microscopy using Ziehl–Neelson stained smears used External Quality Assessment (EQA) to compare the results of various laboratories to a reference laboratory. Misdiagnosed cases were found out using EQA, and an association with other parameters of the same lab such as smear quality, infrastructure, materials used, etc. was established [19]. Such methods can help in identifying the areas with maximum scope of improvement to increase the diagnostic efficacyof the laboratory.

For quality assurance in clinical diagnosis, peer-review QA committees in various departments of the hospitals can help in analyzing the patient care and management, and further suggest areas of improvement. For example, a study was conducted for misdiagnosis of neurological cases in the Emergency Department (ED) of a tertiary care center. QA review committee of the department analyzed medical records, ED course, and interviewed the physicians. This can help in identifying the common errors along with the ways to avoid them [20]. In clinical settings, there are examples of QA being implemented in an online format also. In Harvard Medical School, Boston, an online QA database was developed for Radiology that allowed the staff to submit cases with appropriate imaging for the review. A Quality Management Team (QMT) was also formed that was responsible for assigning a reviewer for each submitted case, as well as for the final review of the case. This method, being computerized, enabled easier monitoring of trends in diagnostic errors, as compared to an offline format. Additionally, this also enabled in finding ways how better training and quality improvement projects can be initiated for the various sources of error [21].

In the case of life-threatening disorders, at least two confirmatory diagnostic tests should be mandatorily done and for particular disorders, certain tests should be considered as the gold standard like RT-PCR for COVID-19. QA implementation in a diagnostic facility can also enhance the diagnostic efficacy along with developing an effective and precise treatment strategy based on the clinical phenotype. Therefore, academic implementation of QA in clinical diagnosis can enhance the overall image of the Institute by minimizing the chances of misdiagnosis of disease, increasing transparency and reproducibility of the diagnostic results.

8.3 Scientific Misconduct: A Lesson from the History

Misconduct in research is not a new topic of discussion. There have been various incidents in the past where misconduct in research was reported and led to dire consequences. One such incidence was the discovery of STAP cells by a Japanese researcher. She claimed that she had discovered an easy way to produce stimulus-triggered acquisition of pluripotency (STAP) cells that can be used to grow tissues. This was apparently considered a path-breaking discovery in the scientific community. She published her discovery in an esteemed journal. Within a few days of this publication, allegations of fraud started emerging on social media platforms. The reported images had been doctored and the text in the papers also appeared to be plagiarized [22]. Her Professor proposed retraction of the pertaining papers and told her to reproduce the experiments, followed by an investigation launched by RIKEN to identify the misconduct and falsification of data generation. It was later found that the images in the paper were from her thesis work and these were two independent scientific works. RIKEN found her guilty of scientific misconduct [23]. She was not able to reproduce her data and it was difficult to verify her poorly kept records. The publications were retracted [24, 25]. Her supervisor was so overwhelmed by the accusation that he committed suicide. This was indeed a heartbreaking incident that has resulted from carelessness in research.

Data fabrication is often done by students during research activities. An Australian researcher also had to retract her papers from esteemed journals related to a clinical trial of Ramipril, which is a drug for hypertension. Later, she admitted to the fabrication of data pertaining to records of the patients [26]. Another Professor working on Cancer research from the Anderson Cancer Centre, University of Texas, MD had to retract publications after fraud was detected in his papers related to Curcumin in cancer [27]. Sometimes, the researchers mislabel their research work, such as lanes in gels. In one of the incidents a former postdoctoral fellow at St. Jude Children's Research Hospital was found to have falsified an image and mislabeled gels, as a result, the papers were retracted from reputed journals including the Journal of Cell Biology and from Molecular and Cellular Biology [28]. Sometimes, the researchers also steal ideas from published work and use them to publish their own [29]. Later on, he was found guilty and his NIH funding was stripped off.

Documentation of results in a doctored fashion is one of the major problems in the research fraternity. The researchers do not keep records of their experimental work, which is a prompt violation of the guidelines of federal research. A cancer researcher at Ohio State University was made to retract his work after an investigation found the falsification of the data without documentation of research data [30]. Consequently, such allegations on researcher/research groups could lead to a ban from publication and receiving grants from funding agencies, if proven guilty. Such was the case of a former associate professor of Ophthalmology at Harvard University Medical School who was found to have fabricated the grants and publications. He was barred from receiving any funding from NIH for the next 10 years [31]. A scientist was found to tamper the experiments to achieve desired results, like it was done by a former assistant professor of biomedical sciences at Iowa State University. Herein, he was working on an AIDS vaccine, and to achieve desirable results he spiked the rabbit blood with the human antibody. He, later on, agreed to all the charges and accepted 5 years imprisonment and returned the funding to NIH [32]. One astounding incident was reported in South Korea where a former professor created fake mail IDs to peer review his own articles [33]. Importantly, compliance to informed consent rules may be overlooked which might have serious implications. Two recently published articles regarding COVID-19 that gained much importance when they were published had to be eventually retracted. The paper citing the efficacy of hydroxychloroquine (HCQ) in treating COVID-19 was retracted from Lancet after the data was found non-reasonable [34]. Another paper was published in NEJM that refuted that those who have been taking ACE inhibitors and ARBs had increased mortality due toCOVID-19. This retraction was due to similar reasons [35]. Falsification of data, reporting the experiments that have not been done, and data forging are common scientific misconduct practices. Students also practice the fabrication of references while writing a paper. They do not read the paper but cite them in the bibliography to meet the demand of a certain number of references as a given guideline by a journal. A multicenter 5-year randomized clinical trial was published in NEJM in 2013, showing a Mediterranean Diet's preventive effect on severe Cardiovascular events implying that the diet was solely responsible for the results, which gained much popularity and was later retracted on grounds of improper randomization among the groups [36]. An anesthesiologist, J B Carlisle investigated several randomized controlled trials across various journals, and he found problems in 5087 trials, including this study [37]. It was revised in 2018, and the results still showed a beneficial effect of the Mediterranean diet but not with as much certainty [36].

In academics, plagiarism is also being practiced while writing a paper and all scientific journals condemn it. Plagiarism refers to borrowing somebody's idea without attribution and rephrasing it in their own words without giving proper citation [38, 39]. It is also defined as the theft of intellectual property. Textual plagiarism is one of the most common plagiarisms found in the scientific field. There are many ways of plagiarism, first and foremost is copying directly, copying ideas and passing it as their own, and also translation of some work which was reported previously in some other language. The incidence of plagiarism has increased in recent years and steps are being taken by academia to curb this problem. As the problem arises because of failure to cite the references, Journals recommend a particular style of citing them. There are many software which help in detecting it and the penalty for it varies from institution to institution. Universities like Stanford, Yale, U.C Berkeley, Massachusetts Institute of Technology (MIT), University of Cambridge, Oxford University, etc. have their own guidelines to handle plagiarism. It also extends to self-plagiarism where authors attempt to publish at two or more different journals with the same data or publish the same results in different language journals. If a journal is having its own policy to curb plagiarism, it should be clearly stated in the author guidelines [40]. Predatory publishing is also on the rise and may promote plagiarism. The term "predatory" was first used by J. Beall, to refer to certain journals, which do not have a proper peer review process in place and maybe quick to publish articles in order to make money, by taking advantage of the open access publishing model [41]. Some of these journals have also been indexed in PubMed, hence, this carries a risk of corrupting the quality of scientific literature, and may also promote plagiarism [42]. These were some examples of scientific misconduct that commonly occur in research. Ensuring Quality assurance at various steps of conducting research can prevent the conflicts generated at later stages.

8.4 Quality Assurance During Formulation of the Research Question

Data is considered of appropriate quality when it lacks an uncertainty and does not exceed the variability and uncertainty when it is considered as of inadequate quality [43]. Beginning from the inception of the research idea after rigorous literature search and further refining it with PI expertise, it is warranted to secure its integrity and possible conflict generation in the research field [44] During this initial stage of research idea genesis, it is likely that a researcher will go through an extensive literature search to explore the novelty of the research, innovation, and its translational implication for societal benefits along with its commercial benefits. Once a decision has been made regarding the novelty of the research question, it needs to be protected from any further duplication or false claim by another research group. To avoid it, the copyright for an idea can be attained on time by producing justifiable documents. It would also be useful to secure such research ideas to publish them online to further strengthen the research, and to avoid any future research conflict. Usually, to address a research question, funding is required and there are many funding agencies that support research, once a grant application is accepted [45]. However, the idea can be copied and two or more research groups can claim the idea as their own. It is also demanding to secure such research ideas to publish online to further strengthen to avoid any research conflict. Conclusively, the copyright of the grant can further support the credibility that the true claimants will be granted financial support from the funding organization.

8.5 Quality Assurance in Research Data Generation

Research needs a series of experiments and steps which must be followed to arrive at a proper conclusion. The research should strictly adhere to ethical standards. There are seven points to ensure that the clinical research is ethical, which are:

1. Research must lead to enhancement of knowledge or benefit one's health.
2. It should be valid scientifically.
3. Participants' selection should be unbiased and fair.
4. Knowledge to society and benefits should overpower the risks.
5. Review of the research should be done by unaffiliated individuals who may recommend to continue or terminate it.
6. Informed consent should be taken from the subjects.
7. Privacy and well-being of the researchers [46]

Before conducting research, it is mandatory to take ethical approval from the institute. The guidelines may vary from one institute to the other and there can be different committees like animal ethical, stem cell ethical, and ethical board for research on human subjects, which after a careful reviewing process provide the approval to the research study. Research also involves data collection and analysis of the data. Data is collected in both scientific and nonscientific studies. Surveying the population, administering questionnaires and performing experiments are ways by which data can be generated. Uniformity should be maintained for all types of data collection to avoid person-to-person variations. Master schedules help in the planning of activities and also in keeping a track of the experiments being performed in a lab. MS should be prepared carefully and should contain all the necessary information related to the study like the nature of the study, date of initiation of the study, current study status, sponsor identity, details of the study director, and the final report status. Master schedules can still be modified for the suitability of the study [47]. Master schedules help in streamlining the activities. MS should be strictly followed and any deviation should be noted. Standard operating protocols are also required to prevent any deviance from the standard procedures. SOPs help in increasing the reproducibility of accumulated data. Maintenance and calibration of laboratory equipment [48] are also integrative parameters in the research domain to avoid the false generation of data. SOPs mainly help to perform the experiments in a planned and defined way. In the future, if a dispute arises regarding the timeline and performance of an experiment, then records of SOPs, procedures and other entries can act as a protective shield to avoid false allegations and worthless claiming. SOPs are documents that specify procedures that must be followed to assure the quality, credibility, and integrity of study data [49]. They also decrease person-to-person variations in the data, which can cause a conflict regarding the experimental outcome. Data Recording Sheets are equally beneficial to prevent any doubt regarding data collection and experiments. DRSs help in keeping data records of the experiments performed and mention the date of performing them (refer to Chap. 5). Appropriate steps need to be followed initially and during the whole process of data generation to avoid any conflicts. Data should be entered carefully in the electronic copies and validated from time to time. Maintaining log entries in logbooks for use of instruments, chemicals, and reagents act as evidence that the researcher has performed the experiments. It also helps in keeping a record of the material, which makes the process easier for future experimenters by providing the details about the usage (refer to Chap. 7). Similarly, log sheets for material purchased from the funding received should be maintained in labs. Log sheets might include log sheets for chemicals, kits, molecular biology reagents, antibodies, plastic ware, etc. The logsheet format may or may not be like the one given below. It should have columns for the name of the material, batch number, catalog number, date of receiving, expiry date, location, quantity date of opening the material followed by a log of its use—how much was used and how much was left, and name and signature of the person using it. Also, raw books can be maintained by students to keep a record of experiments. It should be numbered with layouts of the experiments and the date of performing them. A result folder can also help in keeping records and in preserving them if electronic data is lost. Xerox copies of thermal prints for instrument readings should be taken, as the ink fades away with time. In the case of a questionnaire-based study or a study that involves recruitment of the participants, informed consents should be filled properly and duly signed by the participant, researcher, principal investigator, and witness. It should have details of the risks and benefits of the work. Additionally, it should be clearly mentioned that the subject is participating voluntarily in the study. Participant information sheets should be given to the participants, and details of the study should be explained without concealing anything from them. It should be signed by the Principal Investigator and the researcher who recruits the participant. This can help in avoiding any kind of conflict which may point toward the wrong sample size and misleading data. This is also a proof that participants were informed well ahead of recruiting them in the study and that they have voluntarily participated in the study.

Consent of participants should be treated as of utmost importance to conduct the research ethically [50]. There are a variety of conflicts that arise in academics and research at various stages which are chiefly due to unethical practices, and not following good conduct during research. The case of Jesse Gelsinger is one such case where unethical practice led to the death of the participant. He was the first person to die during the clinical trial of Gene therapy. Despite the risks involved, the researchers did not disclose them and decided to carry on with the procedure which leads to this tragic incident. Later on, the university had to issue a rebuttal. There is no doubt that those participating in Medical research are participating for a noble cause and for the greater good of humanity. Hence, experiments should be conducted ethically. Research malpractice is found in many Institutes, universities, and corporate settings. Compromising with the life of the research subjects should not be encouraged at any cost [51]. Also, misreporting the research data is highly unacceptable. There are many instances in history where researchers/scientists adopt unfair means to tamper the data so it meets the standards of journals for publication. Later on, such publications are retracted and it often brings a bad reputation to the institute and the researchers.

Also, plagiarism should be kept in check and strictly avoided. This can be done with the help of anti-plagiarism websites like www.turnitin.com etc. Plagiarism can be of many types like:

- Verbatim—Using someone else's words without acknowledging them
- Mosaic—Not copying exact words, but mixing own words with someone else's ideas

- Paraphrasing—Rephrasing someone else's words or ideas without citing references
- Self-plagiarism—Publishing own prepublished data
- Cyber plagiarism—Copying and downloading research papers from the internet without citations
- Image plagiarism—Use of images and videos without acknowledging the source [52]

Many committees governing research and Journals have policies for anti-plagiarism. Examples include the University Grants Commission (UGC) guidelines and regulations to avoid the menace of plagiarism in higher education (www.ugc.ac.in). If detected during the initial stages, it leads to rejection and after publishing, a retraction of the publication. It can also lead to serious consequences sometimes. Validation of data is another important step in quality assurance which must be done either by the internal or external validators. Validation from external expertise is mostly preferred, to secure additional transparency toward the absence of bias of the data and results. Once validation is done, the final step of ensuring quality must be followed [53].

8.6 Quality Assurance and Preventing Conflicts During Research Data Presentation

Data should be presented in the most intelligible form. Data is ultimately presented in the form of Publications and Patents [54]. Here, most conflicts arise due to discrepancies between the authors and inventors. Discrepancies can be regarding ownership of the data, representation of the data and the contribution of each author/inventor. To avoid such conflicts, manuscripts should be carefully written and publication agreement form should be filled simultaneously regarding authorship contributions and should be signed by the contributors to avoid any conflicts (Fig. 8.1). There are guidelines given by International Committee of Medical Journal Editors (ICMJE) that must be fulfilled to become an author of a paper.

These are the four basic criteria:

1. Contribution to design and concept of the work, acquisition analysis, and interpreting the data
2. Drafting and critical revision of the work
3. Final approval
4. Agreement to the accountability of work regarding the integrity of the work [55]

Conflicts are also generated when the author making a major contribution is not named while publishing. Hence, the declaration of conflicts of interest becomes important. At a later stage, conflicts are generated at the time of peer review when the editor opines in a suspicious manner giving extremely positive reviews to be included in the research paper's author list. This can be checked by transparency in the review process and blind reviewing which is usually done by many Journals.

Restricted Circulation Photocopy Prohibited

Neuroscience Research Lab
Department of Neurology
Post Graduate Institute of Medical Education and Research

Publication Agreement Form

We, all the authors, declare that the manuscript does not contain any material or information that may be unlawful, defamatory, fabricated or plagiarized. We also certify that the paper is prepared according to the 'Instructions of Authors. We declare that this manuscript has not been submitted elsewhere for publication and none of us have competitive and/or financial interest with this manuscript and have read the manuscript and agreed to authorship as it is presented.

We are not aware of any other potential author who worked towards this paper but was neither excluded from authorship nor aware of any authors here who have been given place in authorship sequence that was not involved in drafting, conceptualization or operationalization of this study or review. We also realize that the title of the paper may change with resubmission and approve of the same in anticipation. We realize that authorship is not synonymous with inventor ship.

Title:

Type of Manuscript: ______________________________

Publishing Journal: ______________________________

Corresponding Author:	Co-author 1:
Name:	Name:
Author's contribution:	Author's contribution:
Affiliation:	Affiliation:
Contact:	Contact:
Email:	Email:
Signature	Signature
Date:____________ Place: ______________	Date:____________ Place: ______________

PGIMER Neuroscience Research Lab

Fig. 8.1 Publication agreement form and inventorship form in a patent application must also be maintained and recorded in GLP compliance laboratory by QA officer with Study Director and PI

Financial conflicts of interest also arise while conducting research. There are many such incidents where the investigators have fabricated the research data, where the investigators had considerable financial interests [56]. In the Journal Lancet, a study was published in 1998, which established a link between developmental disorders in children and immunization with MMR vaccine which was later retracted in 2010, mentioning that "several elements are incorrect" [57] The anti-vaccination movement in some countries was fueled by this research, where the author had undeclared financial conflicts of interest as he had received financial benefits from parents who had pressed charges against the vaccine manufacturer [58]. This example shows how fraudulent research can affect public health in general, as many parents eventually became reluctant to get their children vaccinated. Hence, during a research study, financial interests should not be concealed. That is why it is in the journals' policy to receive a statement where authors declare their conflicts if any.

8.7 Intellectual Property and Conflicts

The area of Intellectual property (IP) is most infested with conflicts and needs careful consideration. Intellectual property is defined as the yield of human intellect. The most commonly recognized intellectual properties include copyrights, patents, trademarks, etc. Intellectual property rights (IPR) are defined as ideas, inventions, and expressions of creativity on the basis of which status of the IPR can be conferred to it for a certain period of time. IPR confers exclusive rights to the creators of the said property so that they can gain commercial benefits from the invention. IPR protects the investment, money, time, and efforts of the inventor [59]. IPR is granted for patents, industrial designs, trademarks, and geographical indications. They need to satisfy certain conditions to qualify as IP, for example, a patent should satisfy the following conditions [60]:

- Novelty
- Industrial application
- Non-obviousness

Trademarks refer to any features of shape, pattern, configuration, or colors applied to a product. Trademarks may also refer to any mark name and logo. Trademarks are eligible for selling, buying, and licensing. Copyrights refer to ideas and can be applied to literary, music, drama, artist, cinematography work, audiotapes, and computer software. Geographical indicators help in identifying goods originating in a country or a territory where their origin is attributable. For example, India has Banaresi sarees, Italy has Parmesan as protected GI and a trademark [61]. In academics, copyrights and patents are more important. Patents are granted for a product or a process. According to the patent act of 1970, it is granted for a period of 14 years for a product, but for a process related to a drug or food, it is granted for a period of 7 years. A patent can be considered as a publication and also as a legal document. The procedure of filing for a patent includes filing a patent application before it is made available to the public, submitting the manuscript for publication and getting it published [62]. For economic benefits of companies, patents, and publications, it shows a reverse trend. There has been a decrease in the profitability of publications in the last 3 decades. In the 1980s, the addition of one publication to the company's stock increased its value by US$6,00,000. However, from 2000 to 2006 the market value of the company has fallen by US$500,000 for each publication. However, for patents, the reverse trend is observed for the company's stock [63]. There has been a shift from publications to patents in large corporations as the knowledge accredited to scientific research is less valued than technical knowledge (Patents).

The right to claim patents was given to universities in order to provide an incentive to the researchers to develop something resourceful from their work [64]. On one hand, a university or academic institution is expected to encourage research that aids in innovation and contributes to society's economic and overall development. There have been efforts to promote this by considering patents and commercialization to be a factor for merit and career advancement in academic institutes [65]. However, on the downside, the academic community may have started focusing more on commercialization and profits as opposed to basic scientific research [64]. Patents have to be claimed before the discoveries and research are revealed to the scientific community and the public, which may delay scientific progress, as a result. An increased incidence of conflicts is also a result of this. There has been a dispute regarding the patent claim of CRISPR genome editing system between two universities, the University of California and The Broad Institute of Harvard and MIT, and the companies who wish to develop a product out of it are not able to approach an academic institution for the same reason [64]. This, in turn, hampers the development of products that can benefit society.Patent infringements can have many repercussions as was in the case of Teva and Sun Pharmaceuticals against Protonix's active ingredient pantoprazole. The dispute originated when the above said companies launched the drug with pantoprazole as its active ingredient preempting the expiry date in 2011. This led to around 60% decline in Pfizer's sales. In 2010 Teva and Sun Pharma were ordered to take this drug down from the market. Their claim for the patent of the widely popular drug Protonix was also obviously rejected. Both the pharma companies were asked to settle the dispute by paying $1.6 billion and $550 million respectively to Pfizer [66]. Another patent infringement dispute was between Centocor and Abbot Laboratories (2009). It was alleged by Centocor that a drug called Humira marketed by Abbot Laboratories has done patent infringement. Their argument was that Humira resembled the Centocor drug called Remicade. A district court jury agreed to this and awarded Centocor compensation. Although later, the decision was reversed on appeal by CAFC on the grounds that the language used for patenting was vague and did not meet the requirements to be considered effective [66]. Steps that need to be followed when applying for a patent are:

- File the patent application with the government, for example, United States Patent and Trademark Office (USPTO)—and check whether it is novel.
- Take the assistance of an attorney to avoid any monetary and time loss.
- Ascertain which type of patent is required. For example—product, process, design etc.
- File a provisional patent application.
- Collect information for a final application consisting of a detailed description of the patent including abstract, background, details, and conclusion. It should also outline the scope of the patent.
- Review the application to prevent any rejections.
- Actively respond to the examiner assigned to your patent application [67].

Once the patent expires, it is no longer protected and would be available in the public domain. It can then be exploited, and which would not count as an infringement. Patents are territorial in nature and are applicable in the country where it was applied. The right to take action against those who infringe remains with the owner of the patent (Licensing of a patent) and is done according to TCs. The patent owner may give a third party right for selling, using, and making the patented invention in return for royalty payments. This is usually due to the absence of facilities for manufacturing and reduction of the total cost. Currently, there is no universal system to grant patents. Hence, the patents cannot be universal [68]. But, if someone wants to apply patent which is applicable in different countries or worldwide, filing an international application under Patent Cooperation Treaty (PCT), administered by World Intellectual Property Organisation (WIPO) can be done. This can be a straightforward approach rather than filing in separate countries. However, to enhance the transparency and auditability of data, many agencies provide accreditation for quality assurance like the Quality Council of India (QCI). Getting an accreditation certificate from one of the constituent boards of QCI can also ensure quality. National Accreditation Board for Testing and Calibration Laboratories (NABL) provides accreditation to testing laboratories, calibration laboratories, medical laboratories, proficiency testing providers, and reference material providers. NABL is a signatory to ILAC arrangements as APAC Mutual Recognition Arrangements (MRA). International arrangements of such type help facilitate the acceptability of test results and help calibrate between countries to which MRA partners represent [69, 70]. Hence, NABL or GLP accreditation (and following the procedure as per norms) and timely review by external expertise are required to enhance the authenticity, reproducibility, and transparency of the data. The process to get NABL accreditation is outlined in Fig. 8.2.

The CAB must make all the pending payments to NABL. The accreditation is given for a period of 2 years. Annual surveillance is conducted by NABL after a

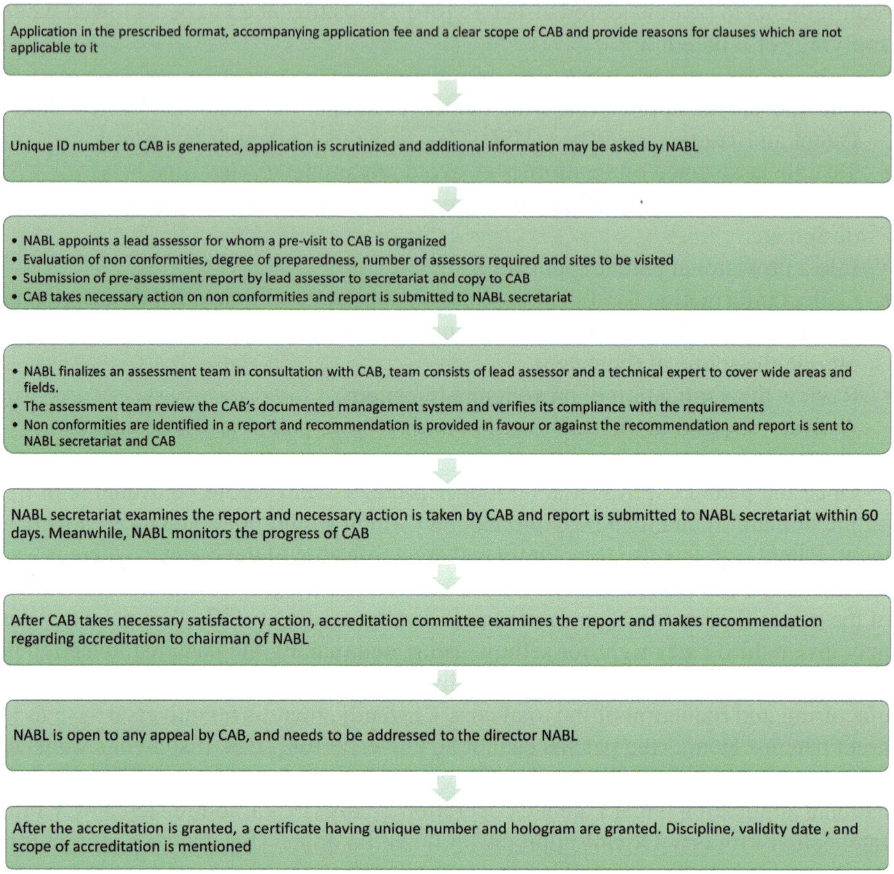

Fig. 8.2 A process to get NABL accreditation of clinical laboratory. Periodic calibration and maintenance of records under the purview of QA is the primary foundation of the same

period of 1 year to check compliance with the requirements. Reassessment is done after 2 years. CAB is required to apply 6 months prior to the expiry of the accreditation so that it can be continued [69].

Food and Drug Administration (FDA) is an agency of the United States Department of Health and Human Services. In addition to its health-promoting policies, it ensures the quality of a drug by an in-built system to scrutinize it at various stages for its safety and efficacy. Center for Drug Evaluation and Research (CDER) monitors this system. Drug companies who seek approval from FDA must test it first for safety and efficacy. Then the company sends data to CDER as evidence that the drug is safe and effective. A team of CDER physicians, pharmacologists, chemists, statisticians, and other scientists review the data that the company provides. If the review is independent and unbiased, and benefits outweigh the risks, the drug is approved for marketing. The center itself does not test the drugs but conducts the research in areas of drug quality, safety, and effectiveness standard. The approval of any drug follows a structured framework [71]:

- Target and present treatments are analyzed.
- Risks and benefits from clinical data are assessed.
- Strategies for risk management are formulated.

A laboratory must comply with GLP to improve the reliability, back traceability, and credibility of the data. National GLP Compliance Monitoring authority established by the Department of Science and Technology, Govt. of India provides GLP certification to Industries, test facilities, and laboratories dealing with Industrial chemicals, Pharmaceuticals (Human and Veterinary), Agrochemicals, Cosmetics Products, Food/Feed Additives, and Medical devices. India is a member of Mutual acceptance of data in the OECD working group, which makes data generated in nonclinical laboratory settings (health and safety studies complied to GLP) acceptable in 36 OECD countries and six non-OECD countries adhering to MAD. The demand for GLP compliant laboratories is increasing, and to cater to this need NGCMA has 17 GLP inspectors from different government institutes, universities, and laboratories. Certification from GLP is voluntary in nature:

- Apply in the prescribed application form of NGCMA.
- Pre-inspection is done.
- Final inspection is done.
- The final decision report is sent to the chairman/GLP authority regarding GLP certification.
- GLP Certification is valid for 3 years and surveillance is conducted after 18 months from the date of certification.
- Inspection for recertification is done during the 3rd year.

NGCMA also organizes workshops and training for sensitizing the research fraternity for GLP [72]. The researchers should always pay utmost attention to research/academics at every stage to maintain transparency and reproducibility of the data. Complying with GLP is one of the ways to ensure it [73]. Also, maintaining GLP with the help of QA personnel is important. QA officers can help in better management in conducting research. This will not only help in increasing the liability of the research outcome but also help in smoothly conducting the research activities in an organized and integrative manner.

8.8 Role of Quality Assurance Officer in Ensuring Quality and Avoiding Conflicts in Academics

As discussed above, the huge responsibility of a QA officer is evident in all aspects of research activities, and it can help ensure and attain optimum quality, avoid bias toward the results, provide credit to the personnel for their contribution (in the form of publication and owning inventorship in the patent application) in research practice. Following are some of the duties performed by the QA officer in a scientific laboratory.

8.8.1 At Experimental and Academic Levels

1. Master schedules are usually submitted to a QA person who has the duty to see whether it has been followed.
2. To issue the DRS timely to the researchers for smooth conduct of experiments as per the timeline. QA also has to ensure that the DRS is filled correctly and is verified by the study director, followed by submission to QA personnel. This will ensure the further maintenance of the records which are devoid of tampering of data recording and also to enhance the back traceability of the experiments, even in the absence of the researcher.
3. To keep observatory records of calibration and maintenance of the laboratory instruments, so that experiments do not suffer and the results are reliable. QA can also direct the associated personnel to conduct timely calibration of an instrument by informing the study director.
4. A GLP laboratory usually maintains logsheets of chemicals, reagents, and instruments. A QA person can keep an observatory of records of their timely and proper completion. This further ensures quality in the research domain.
5. To submit monthly reports to the study director regarding the use/disuse, expiry status of chemicals and reagents.
6. To prepare a report on basic laboratory facilities, electricity and water supply and to submit it to the study director to take or instructions for further action, if needed.

Study-based inspection is also desirable from a QA officer to ensure whether the reported experiments (as per the MS of the respective researcher) are being performed correctly and the record is being kept. At the end of the month, a QA report needs to be generated to make the researchers aware of the record of the work done and suggestions of the QA/PI for the betterment of research protocols in academics and also to get credit to the researchers.

8.8.2 To Secure the Inception of the Research Idea

It is a common practice in academic research to steal a research idea and to take credit for it. Hence, QA personnel can contribute by maintaining the records of the timeline of data generated by the researcher, and further conceptualization of the research question(s) based on the outcome of prior research. Proper documentation of experiments, publications (by maintaining publication agreement form based on contribution), grant writing and their prior registration (if any), and getting the copyrights of an idea can promote and secure the research idea and prevent it from getting falsely claimed. In the case of a collaboration, adequate documentation of the credit/sharing based on the amount of contribution must be done by the QA personnel before moving for international and national collaborations. Collaboration approval from the parent Institute along with contribution-based credit must be well uttered and preserved as a record with QA personnel. Formulation and amendments in the research question must also be documented on time. The duties of QA personnel in a GLP laboratory are summarized in Fig. 8.3.

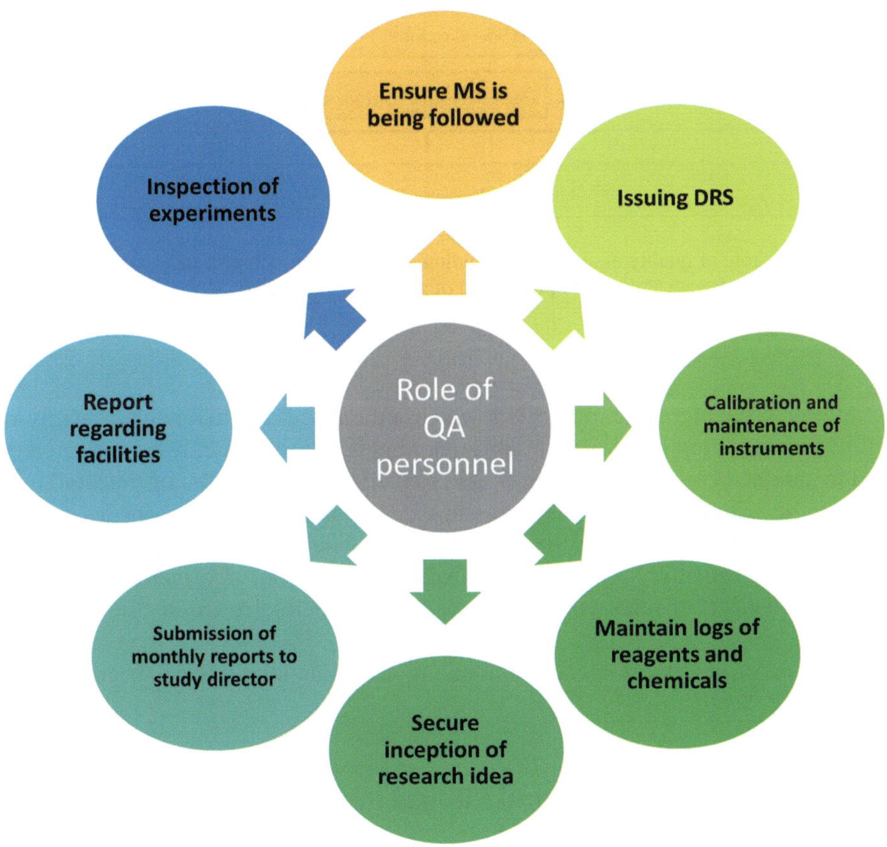

Fig. 8.3 The duties of QA personnel in a GLP laboratory to ensure quality assurance concerning data generation and research

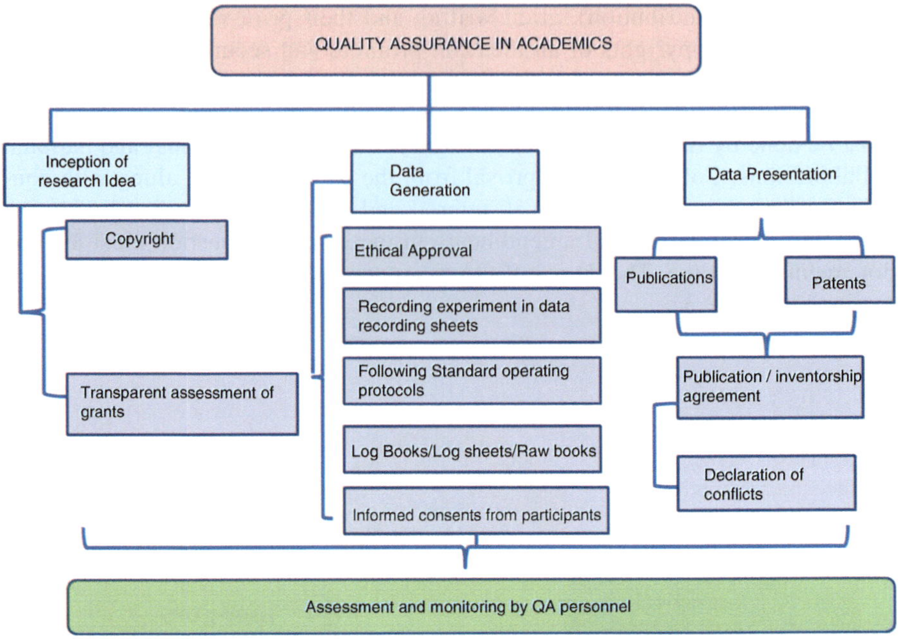

Fig. 8.4 The role of quality assurance in avoiding academic conflicts and ensuring reproducibility, reliability, back traceability, and prevention of academic misconduct

Master schedule, DRS, and SOPs which are created and maintained merely to fulfill the regulatory requirements are monotonous and tiresome. If they are created and maintained casually, then it may lead to ineffective utilization of time and may burden the administration. Quality assurance should not just be considered as a choice but must be followed mandatorily in research to avoid any conflicts and maintained creatively. It not only improves the quality but also increases the reliability of data. It ensures well-planned and reproducible research free from any conflicts.

The role of quality assurance in avoiding academic conflicts has been summarized in Fig. 8.4.

8.9 Future Directions and Clinical Implications

QA in academics can play a crucial role to understand the risk, procedure, deviations, and its immediate amendment in the clinical and research setup to improve the quality. QA's risk assessment and fact-based remarks can provide the critical inputs to update and amend the established conventions, assumptions and enable us to prepare a framework to channelize the various procedures and activities in academics. Therefore, it is demanded to encourage the efforts of QA in academics and to publish those critical remarks and inputs in respective SOPs, procedure in addition to any deviation. QA's quality assessment in clinical research and nonclinical research can significantly improve the diagnostic efficacy and translation of research outcome but requires a new law that mandates GLP implementation mandatory for all research labs. Copyright conflicts, false claims, and fabrication of data which is imperative in active labs, can be dealt by QA in related clinical and research setup. This will also provide the substrate to channelize the various activities at the level of academics (collaboration, patent, or false allegation of recruitment procedure) and can enable us to provide the framework to prepare SOPs, guidelines, and respective amendments at institutional, national, and international levels.

8.10 Conclusion

Quality assurance is required not only in manufacturing units and corporates but also in academics and research. QA helps to avoid any conflicts generated at various stages of research. There are many academic misconduct like fabrication of data, copying data, unethical research, obscuring information from the participants, ignoring ethical guidelines, plagiarism, non-reproducible research, financial and publishing disagreements, leading to academic conflicts. These are mainly due to a lack of proper documentation, like not following QA. Assurance of Quality at various steps of research during the formulation of research question, during data generation, and data presentation in the form of patents and publications can prevent many of these conflicts. Documents like SOPs, DRSs help in increasing the reproducibility of research. Validation of data and records, maintenance of log sheets, instrument logbooks and complying with ethical guidelines, anti-plagiarism policies, obtaining copyrights for ideas, grants, etc., providing participant information sheet to subjects, obtaining informed consents from subjects are equally important for ethical research. Publication agreement forms should be mandatorily filled before submission of a manuscript in the journal and all conflicts must be stated in a declaration statement. Following GLP which ensures the prevention of academic conflicts, whether accusations inspired by personal benefits or jealousy. GLP not only helps in defending against false accusations but also ensures quality in research, which can have greater applicability and can benefit mankind.

Acknowledgment We are grateful to Prof. Sudhir Srivastava for his valuable comments on various aspects of QA responsibilities in academics.

References

1. ISO 9000:2005, Clause 3.2.10.
2. CNBC. House investigation finds Boeing's 737 Max was 'marred' by technical problems, lack of transparency [Internet]. 2020. https://www.cnbc.com/2020/03/06/house-investigation-finds-boeings-737-max-was-marred-by-technical-problems-lack-of-transparency.html. Accessed 8 Dec 2020.
3. BBC. California wildfires sparked minutes after electrical failure [Internet]. 2019. https://www.bbc.com/news/world-us-canada-50172228. Accessed 8 Dec 2020.

4. Vogel G. Microbiome researcher accused of sexual misconduct. Science. 2020;367(6480):837–8.
5. Irish BJ. The varieties of early modern envy and jealousy: the case of obtrectation. Mod Philol. 2019;117(1):115–26.
6. Reynolds J, Kizito J, Ezumah N, Mangesho P, Allen E, Chandler C. Quality assurance of qualitative research: a review of the discourse. Health Res Policy Syst. 2011;9(1):43.
7. Zavalina OL, Phillips M, Tarver HS. Quality assurance and evaluation of change for patent metadata. Proc Assoc Inf Sci Technol. 2017;54(1):842–3.
8. Kaushal MS, Tyagi R, Banik A, Battu MP, Mehra MP, Sharma NK, Sharma MK, Anand A. A unique data validation process by internal and external quality assurance system aimed to combat research malpractice. Int J Sci Res. 2019;8(8)
9. Hyland K. Self-citation and self-reference: credibility and promotion in academic publication. J Am Soc Inf Sci Technol. 2003;54(3):251–9.
10. Mishra S, Fegley BD, Diesner J, Torvik VI. Self-citation is the hallmark of productive authors, of any gender. PLoS One. 2018;13(9):e0195773.
11. Kulkarni AV, Aziz B, Shams I, Busse JW. Author self-citation in the general medicine literature. PLoS One. 2011;6(6):e20885.
12. Urlings MJ, Duyx B, Swaen GM, Bouter LM, Zeegers MP. Citation bias and other determinants of citation in biomedical research: findings from six citation networks. J Clin Epidemiol. 2020; https://doi.org/10.1016/j.jclinepi.2020.11.019.
13. Haghighat M, Hayatdavoudi J. How hot are hot papers? The issue of prolificacy and self-citation stacking. Scientometrics. 2020;17:1–4.
14. Moiwo JP, Tao F. The changing dynamics in citation index publication position China in a race with the USA for global leadership. Scientometrics. 2013;95(3):1031–50.
15. Liu X, Zhang J, Guo C. Full-text citation analysis: a new method to enhance scholarly networks. J Am Soc Inf Sci Technol. 2013;64(9):1852–63.
16. Sciencemag.org. India needs more transparency in its COVID-19 vaccine trials, critics say [Internet]. 2020. https://www.sciencemag.org/news/2020/11/india-needs-more-transparency-its-covid-19-vaccine-trials-critics-say. Accessed 8 Dec 2020.
17. Matson PL. Internal quality control and external quality assurance in the IVF laboratory. Hum Reprod. 1998;13 Suppl 4:156–65.
18. WHO. Content sheet 10-1: overview of external quality assessment (EQA). https://www.who.int/ihr/training/laboratory_quality/10_b_eqa_contents.pdf
19. Desalegn DM, Kitila KT, Balcha HM, Gebeyehu CS, Kidan YW, Amare K, et al. Misdiagnosis of pulmonary tuberculosis and associated factors in peripheral laboratories: a retrospective study, Addis Ababa, Ethiopia. BMC Res Notes. 2018;11(1):291.
20. Dubosh NM, Edlow JA, Lefton M, Pope JV. Types of diagnostic errors in neurological emergencies in the emergency department. Diagnosis (Berl). 2015;2(1):21–8.
21. Kruskal JB, Yam CS, Sosna J, Hallett DT, Milliman YJ, Kressel HY. Implementation of online radiology quality assurance reporting system for performance improvement: initial evaluation. Radiology. 2006;241:518–27.
22. The Guardian. What pushes scientists to lie? The disturbing but familiar story of Haruko Obokata [Internet]. 2015. https://www.theguardian.com/science/2015/feb/18/haruko-obokata-stap-cells-controversy-scientists-lie. Accessed 8 Dec 2020.
23. Newsweek.com. Haruko Obokata, who claimed stem cell breakthrough, found guilty of scientific misconduct [Internet]. 2014. https://www.newsweek.com/haruko-obokata-who-claimed-stem-cell-breakthrough-found-guilty-scientific-239000. Accessed 8 Dec 2020.
24. Obokata H, Sasai Y, Niwa H, Kadota M, Andrabi M, Takata N, et al. Retracted article: Bidirectional developmental potential in reprogrammed cells with acquired pluripotency. Nature. 2014;505(7485):676–80.
25. Obokata H, Wakayama T, Sasai Y, Kojima K, Vacanti MP, Niwa H, et al. Retracted article: Stimulus-triggered fate conversion of somatic cells into pluripotency. Nature. 2014;505(7485):641–7.

26. BBC. Australian scientist admits fabricating research data [Internet]. 17 Sept 2015. https://www.bbc.com/news/world-australia-34275648.
27. retractionwatch.com. Cancer journals retract 10 papers, flag 8 more, and apologize for the delay [Internet]. 2015. https://retractionwatch.com/2018/09/04/cancer-journals-retract-10-papers-flag-8-more-and-apologize-for-the-delay/. Accessed 8 Dec 2020
28. The-scientist.com. St. Jude postdoc faked images [Internet]. 2011. https://www.the-scientist.com/news-opinion/st-jude-postdoc-faked-images-42317/. Accessed 8 Dec 2020
29. Washingtonpost.com. NIH accuses biologist of stealing ideas from rival researcher [Internet]. 1989. https://www.washingtonpost.com/archive/politics/1989/07/13/nih-accuses-biologist-of-stealing-ideas-from-rival-researcher/fd8a3122-c461-49d8-bd05-c8b99e930f2d/. Accessed8 Dec 2020
30. the-scientist.com. OSU professor falsified data on eight papers, resigns [Internet]. 2018. https://www.the-scientist.com/the-nutshell/osu-professor-falsified-data-on-eight-papers-resigns-29849. Accessed 8 Dec 2020
31. thedp.com. Prof accepts penalty for past misconduct [Internet]. 2000. https://www.thedp.com/article/2000/11/prof_accepts_penalty_for_past_misconduct. Accessed 8 Dec 2020
32. aaas.org. Scientist pleads guilty to fraud in falsification of HIV vaccine test results [Internet]. 2015. https://www.aaas.org/news/scientist-pleads-guilty-fraud-falsification-hiv-vaccine-test-results. Accessed 8 Dec 2020
33. Chronicle.com. Fake peer reviews, the latest form of scientific fraud, fool journals [Internet]. 2012. https://www.chronicle.com/article/fake-peer-reviews-the-latest-form-of-scientific-fraud-fool-journals/. Accessed 8 Dec 2020
34. Mehra MR, et al. Retraction-hydroxychloroquine or chloroquine with or without a macrolide for treatment of COVID-19: a multinational registry analysis. Lancet. 2020;395(10240):1820. https://www.thelancet.com/journals/lancet/article/PIIS0140-6736(20)31324-6/fulltext
35. Mehra MR, et al. Retraction: cardiovascular disease, drug therapy, and mortality in Covid-19. N Engl J Med. 2020. https://doi.org/10.1056/NEJMoa2007621.
36. Ramón Estruch R, Ros E, Salvadó JS, Covas MI, Corella D, Arós F, et al. Primary prevention of cardiovascular disease with a Mediterranean diet. N Engl J Med. 2018;378(25):e34.
37. Carlisle JB. Data fabrication and other reasons for non-random sampling in 5087 randomised, controlled trials in anaesthetic and general medical journals. Anaesthesia. 2017;72(8):944–52.
38. Pennycook A. Reflecting on borrowed words. Tesol Q. 2016;50(2):480–2.
39. Maurer HA, Kappe F, Zaka B. Plagiarism—a survey. J UCS. 2006;12(8):1050–84.
40. Wame.org. Recommendations on Publication Ethics Policies for Medical Journals [Internet]. 2016. http://www.wame.org/resources/publication-ethics-policies-for-medical-journals/. Accessed 8 Dec 2020
41. Beall J. Predatory publishers are corrupting open access. Nature. 2012;489:179.
42. Manca A, et al. The surge of predatory open-access in neurosciences and neurology. Neuroscience. 2017;353:166–73.
43. Taylor JK. Quality assurance of chemical measurements. Boca Raton, FL: CRC; 1987.
44. Tim Woods MB, Walker I. Quality assurance and quality control of thromboelastography and rotational thromboelastometry: the UK NEQAS for blood coagulation experience. In: Seminars in thrombosis and hemostasis 2010, vol. 36, no. 7, p. 757–63.
45. Lindgreen A, Di Benedetto CA, Verdich C, Vanhamme J, Venkatraman V, Pattinson S, Clarke AH, Khan Z. How to write really good research funding applications. Ind Market Manag. 2019;77:232–9.
46. Emanuel EJ, Wendler D, Grady C. What makes clinical research ethical. JAMA. 2000;283(20):2701–11.
47. Goeke J. The Master Schedule Index. In: Carson P, Dent N, editors. Good clinical, laboratory and manufacturing practices. Cambridge: RSC; 2007.
48. World Health Organization. Good laboratory practice training manual: for the trainee: a tool for training and promoting good laboratory practice (GLP) concepts in disease endemic countries. Accessed 8 Dec 2020

49. Parks AE. Standard operating procedures: one element of a program for compliance with good laboratory practice regulations? In: American Chemical Society symposium series; 1988.
50. Garces A, MacGuire E, Franklin HL, Alfaro N, Arroyo G, Figueroa L, et al. Looking beyond the numbers: quality assurance procedures in the Global Network for Women's and Children's Health Research Maternal Newborn Health Registry. Reprod Health. 2020;17(2):1–8.
51. Sciencehistory.org. The death of Jesse Gelsinger, 20 years later [Internet]. 2019. https://www.sciencehistory.org/distillations/the-death-of-jesse-gelsinger-20-years-later. Accessed 8 Dec 2020
52. Dhammi IK, UlHaq R. What is plagiarism and how to avoid it? Indian J Orthop. 2016;50(6):581–3.
53. Kumar PM. Academic audit and quality assurance in higher education. Int J Manag Technol Soc Sci (IJMTS). 2017;2(2):61–8.
54. Campbell JD, Perry R, Papadopoulos NG, Krishnan J, Brusselle G, Chisholm A, Bjermer L, Thomas M, Van Ganse E, Van Den Berge M, Quint J. The REal Life EVidenceAssessmeNt Tool (RELEVANT): development of a novel quality assurance asset to rate observational comparative effectiveness research studies. Clin Transl Allergy. 2019;9(1):21.
55. Icmje.org. Defining the role of authors and contributors [Internet]. http://www.icmje.org/recommendations/browse/roles-and-responsibilities/defining-the-role-of-authors-and-contributors.html. Accessed 8 Dec 2020
56. Korn D. Conflicts of interest in biomedical research. JAMA. 2000;284(17):2234–7.
57. Wakefield AJ, Murch SH, Anthony A, et al. Ileal-lymphoid-nodular hyperplasia, non-specific colitis, and pervasive developmental disorder in children [retracted in: Lancet. 2010;375(9713):445]. Lancet. 1998;351(9103):637–41.
58. Hussain A, Ali S, Ahmed M, Hussain S. The anti-vaccination movement: a regression in modern medicine. Cureus. 2018;10(7):e2919.
59. Singh DR. Law relating to intellectual property: a complete comprehensive material on intellectual property covering acts, rules, conventions, treaties, agreements, digest of cases and much more. New Delhi: Universal Law Publishing; 2008.
60. Saha CN, Bhattacharya S. Intellectual property rights: an overview and implications in pharmaceutical industry. J Adv Pharm Technol Res. 2011;2(2):88.
61. Ipeg.com. Geographical Indications, the example of Sumbawa Honey [Internet]. 2012. https://www.ipeg.com/geographical-indications/. Accessed 8 Dec 2020
62. baa.no. The advantages of academic patenting [Internet]. 2019. https://baa.no/en/all-articles/the-advantages-of-academic-patenting. Accessed 8 Dec 2020
63. Arora A, Belenzon S, Patacconi A. Papers to patents. Nature. 2017;552(7683):S10.
64. Eisen M. Patents are destroying the soul of academic science [Internet]. 20 Feb 2017. http://www.michaeleisen.org/blog/?p=1981. Accessed 16 Dec 2020
65. Sanbergv PR, Gharib M, Harker PT, Kaler EW, Marchase RB, Sands TD, et al. Changing the academic culture: valuing patents and commercialization toward tenure and career advancement. Proc Natl Acad Sci U S A. 2014;111(18):6542–7.
66. Lawyer-monthly.com. The most damaging patent disputes ever [Internet]. 2020. https://www.lawyer-monthly.com/2020/07/the-most-damaging-patent-disputes-ever/. Accessed 8 Dec 2020
67. Inc.com. How to file a patent in 8 easy steps. [Internet]. 2016. https://www.inc.com/larry-kim/how-to-file-a-patent-in-8-easy-steps.html Accessed 8 Dec 2020
68. wipo.int. Frequently asked questions: patents [Internet]. https://www.wipo.int/patents/en/faq_patents.html. Accessed 8 Dec 2020
69. nabl. FAQ [Internet]. https://nabl-india.org/faq/#8
70. qcin.org. Frequently asked questions [Internet]. 2015. https://www.qcin.org/faq.php. Accessed 8 Dec 2020
71. FDA. Development & approval process | Drugs [Internet]. 2019. https://www.fda.gov/drugs/development-approval-process-drugs. Accessed 8 Dec 2020
72. dst.gov.in. Documents of NGCMA [Internet]. 2020. https://dst.gov.in/documents-ngcma. Accessed 8 Dec 2020
73. Tight M. Research into quality assurance and quality management in higher education. In: Theory and method in higher education research. Emerald; 2020.

Data Fraud and Essence of Data Verifiability

9

Parul Bali, L. V. Simhachalam Kutikuppala, Pramod Avti, and Bikash Medhi

9.1 History

Incidents of data misconduct and fraud have been periodic in the medical science and biomedical research field history. Sincerity, data integrity, and trustworthiness are the ground principles pertaining to any scientific research [1] toward the progression of science and the public perception of scientific results adhering to the basic principles is a must. Any deviation from the principles described above could be regarded as scientific fraud or misconduct [2].

The history of science and research is crammed with some unusual instances with proven or questionable misconduct in science [3]. A few giants in science have been found vulnerable to suspicion of ambiguous practices, including the great Isaac Newton, who is noted for falsifying a bit of data for making people admit much relatively toward his hypotheses [4]. Claudius Ptolemy, a mathematician, geographer, astronomer, and astrologer, wrote several scientific disquisitions suspected of notifying the work concluded by others as his straight observations [5]. An esteemed scientist regarded as a founder of the modern science of genetics raises doubts about selective notification of some results and even data fabrication [6]. Among those mentioned and even furthermore such examples, there might be no

P. Bali · P. Avti
Department of Biophysics, Post Graduate Institute of Medical Education and Research, Chandigarh, India

L. V. S. Kutikuppala
Konaseema Institute of Medical Sciences and Research Foundation, Amalapuram, Andhra Pradesh, India

B. Medhi (✉)
Department of Pharmacology, Post Graduate Institute of Medical Education and Research, Chandigarh, India
e-mail: medhi.bikash@pgimer.edu.in

A. Anand (ed.), *Quality Assurance Implementation in Research Labs*,
https://doi.org/10.1007/978-981-16-3074-3_9

straightforward evidence of fraud generally, but just the statistical proof which remarks the perceived observations to be more misaligned to the actual expected theoretical values, whichever could be appropriate, with a probability of affecting the experimental actual data [7].

A researcher, who published a study notifying an association between "measles, mumps and rubella vaccination" with a syndrome comprising bowel disease and autism in 12 children on February 28, 1998, in the Lancet, after which no evidence of this link is established by many epidemiological studies [8]. Nevertheless, retraction of this study happened in the year 2010 after 12 long years, due to the claims against this study stating the children were attributed consecutively, mentioning that the investigations that were accepted by the local ethics committee were proven to be fabricated [9]. Thereby, this researcher's unethical misconduct generated long-standing damage by diminishing the rates of vaccination and distrust in general among healthcare officials, which happened between 1998 and 2010 [10].

A Japanese anesthesiologist and researcher extensively published his clinical trials by involving the agents which are used in the treatment of postoperative nausea and vomiting. In April 2000, attention was caught through an editorial letter to the Journal of Anaesthesia and Analgesia about the atypical results reported through his papers' clinical trials [11]. Such results of the clinical trials were published over the next 12 years. He was penalized for the fabrication of most of his results in 2012, through a *judicial* statistical analysis of data published by him, which showed that the subjects in this study had not been randomly allocated to the different treatment groups as he claimed [12]. With around 190 retracted papers, he holds the current record for the world's most retracted papers [13].

9.2 Types of Scientific Misconduct: Falsification, Fabrication, Plagiarism, and Deception

Scientific misconduct is defined as fabricating, falsifying, plagiarizing, or practicing any fraudulent methods that deviate seriously through the frequently acceptable practices within the scientific group to propose, conduct, or report research that does not comprise differences in interpreting or honest errors or data judgment [14].

Types of scientific misconduct [15]:

1. Fabrication
2. Falsification
3. Plagiarism
4. Deception

Falsification, Fabrication, and Plagiarism are the most frequent kinds of scientific misconduct, among which the most frequent type of misconduct is Plagiarism. Such incidents of scientific misconduct are collectively called the "Unholy trinity of Scientific Writing" [16].

Fabrication means inventing data or information, involving the creation of new documents of results or data. The most frequently fabricated scientific research records are informed consent forms and patient records [17].

For example, a researcher from Berkeley University who is a doctoral graduate with a political degree attempted the replication that gradually advanced to accusation and retraction of another scientist research paper from the *Science* journal. Another researcher is from UCLA, who is a political science doctoral graduate. With his supervising person, another researcher published a paper in "Science," which found that long-term voters' attitude influences gay marriage that can be identified through personal contact by gay canvassers. This researcher had also forwarded a requisition to uSamp, the same surveying firm that another researcher used to collect the data for his study, and discovered that the other researcher has not at all worked together with uSamp. Furthermore, he fabricated the whole mailing communication with a representative of uSamp. Moreover, this another researcher had also made up the uSamp representative himself potentiating the data fabrication leading to scientific misconduct [18].

Falsification means altering the observed result or existing records of a scientific experiment, ranging from fabricating a bit of data to falsifying the entire experiment [19]. Falsification finally leads to omission or distortion of unwanted results or data. Detection of falsification could be challenging, and if identified the retrospective detection of scientific misconduct can even lead to the retraction of several years of published articles [20]. One common example of falsification can be deliberately intensifying sample size for increasing the reputation and credibility of the study for publishing quickly and easily without performing the actual study [21].

For example, "social psychology" Professor from "Tilburg University," the Netherlands in 2010 holds disrepute for his work's misconduct, indicating the study preparation and designs to be created in compliance with his ideas, without administering the questionnaires used for the study to the subjects. Furthermore, Stapel had also fabricated datasets of his own and shared them with his colleagues, intending for authorship on their papers. Later on, Stapel admitted his misconduct for falsifying the studies records and eventually was released from his position at Tilburg University [22].

Plagiarism refers to copying others' work and then projecting the work as their own without proper indexing and citations. The term "plagiarism" comes from a Latin word, "plagiarius," meaning kidnapper or hijacker [23]. From the World Association of Medical Editors' strict definition, an article or paragraph is said to be plagiarized when 7–11 words overlap with a set of 30 letters or 6 consecutive words of a sentence are copied [24]. It is a bit difficult to detect plagiarism, which is hazardous to the well-being of scientific compositions and literature. The availability of free or open access online journals and easy access to the internet could be chief sources of present-day plagiarism amongst the students, researchers, and faculty of every profession [25]. The knowledgeable reviewers suspect plagiarism through notable expertise and excellence in that specific field. Most of the editorial staff of Journals use electronic plagiarism checks (software) to detect plagiarism [26].

The plagiarized words or sentences can be classified into (a) direct (partial/complete copy of files or text including video or audio recordings without properly acknowledging or recognizing the primary source); (b) self-plagiarism (copying or duplicating text of one's own for their other portion of work); (c) mosaic (acquiring the opinions or ideas through actual sources, few phrases and words and improperly quoting those sources) [27].

For example, a person duplicates the other writer's work for their purpose with no effort toward acknowledging the material. The similarity index is *the degree of match or overlap between the author's work compared to the other sources already existing, such as websites, research articles, and books that are available in the similarity checking tool databases.*

Deception refers to deliberately concealing the conflict of inclusion or interests of some ambiguous sentences or statements purposefully within the research protocols or proposals or any other documents related [21]. For example, suppose one of the authors of a research project submits their teamwork to a journal as a primary author without intimating to the coauthors due to some internal conflicts. In that case, this comes under deception through the concealment of conflicts of interest.

9.3 Types of Manipulation

The manipulation of data representation can be:

1. Manipulation by temptation of image

   Each image presented in a scientific article is a precise representation of what is observed actually from the results. Image quality has some implications depending on the care with which it was obtained and processed [28]. It has been assumed that the repetition of an experiment multiple times is required in order to obtain good quality and consistent image for representation [29]. The temptation of image manipulation may look self-convincing to perform, but if such type of misconduct is identified, it will deprive and puts the career and future of that person at stake and even of his/her colleagues [30].

   For example, using a software-based manipulation tool to manipulate an image of research data by applying purposeful changes to those digital images such as double exposure, changing the brightness, etc., can be damaging.
2. Manipulation of graphs

   Graphs are the major constituents of the scientific language and literature due to their ability to condense and summarize large data sets. These graphs are a symbolic representation for displaying the experimental findings of science and research [31]. For example, the use of percentages as labels on a pie chart can be misleading to the readers when the sample size is small. Further, when the percentages are intentionally increased to show more impactful results, they constitute manipulation of graphs.
3. Manipulation of values

   Manipulation of values refers to purposeful control over the data variables, commonly independent variables. The value of an independent variable that a study participant experiences can be manipulated by the researcher for a purposeful outcome, which even helps to control the external variables [32].

For example, when a person working on psychological stress research, *manipulating the participants' stress levels intentionally to depict high impactful results is regarded as manipulating* values.

9.4 Country-Wise Cases of Data Fraud

According to the latest literature, the article retractions from the Journals had increased by ten times in the last decade and the data fraud accounted for around 60% of all those retractions. The retraction numbers increased exponentially in the current times due to the strict and improved editorial practices and encouragement to the editors by the journals to take the retractions seriously [33]. From the PubMed retractions data between 2008 and 2012, when authors belonging to more than 50 countries were noted as having withdrawn papers. USA is the country to retract most papers followed by China to retract "most papers for plagiarism and duplicate publication." Although the unethical publication procedures and practices can differ from one nation to the other, the duplicate publication and plagiarism rates were found to be the most in Finland and Italy [34].

During 1990–2019, a total of 18,603 retractions discovered from 4289 Journals are found to be associated with 753 publishers (or publishing organizations), and China ranked first amongst "top 15" countries, followed by the USA, India, Japan, and Germany [35].

The authors belonging to China, the USA, and India were found accountable for the highest number of retractions in plagiarism and duplicate publications. The global retraction rates differ from country to country, and foremost authors from low-income countries have a greater probability of retraction concerning plagiarism than the foremost authors from high-income countries. Looking into detail about duplicate publications and plagiarism it reflects poorly on the retraction and publishing practices of that country among multiple countries. Duplicate publications and plagiarism together account for approximately 35% of all the retractions. The incidence of fabricated publications is more common than plagiarism, resulting in more papers being withdrawn because of fabricated publication. Besides, many countries are having duplicate publication retractions than plagiarism retractions [36].

In general, the authors working in countries that have developed appropriate policies and offices to handle and enforce rules against scientific misconduct are likely to have fewer retractions. All the countries need to address the issues of plagiarism and duplication of publication in a regulated manner to ensure ethical research practices. Unethical behaviors among scientists manifest as a breach in publishing ethics and vary between different countries [37].

9.5 Misconduct in Clinical Trials

An increased incidence of misconduct in clinical trials is reported in recent years, and there is a chance of additional undetected or unreported cases. Probable fraud of data that is not recognized through routine on-site monitoring measures can be identified by adopting stringent clinical trial monitoring procedures, thereby improving the overall data quality [38]. Few economic statistical central monitoring procedures must be made as part of the comprehensive data quality assurance programs for early detection of data fraud and other data-related problems and at a correctable point of time during the clinical trial [39].

Most of the Institutions categorize misconduct of research in the clinical trials as a terrible kind of misconduct due to wide-ranging implications and deleterious consequences on the welfare of public and public perception and perspective [40]. Such scientific misconduct requires instant restorative measures. Misconduct in clinical trials is regarded as an offense in contrast to the good practices and ethical principles that are acceptable in the clinical and scientific environment. Procedures and strategies ensuring the data quality in the clinical trials, including the detection and treatment of data fraud are essential and critical to ensuring clinical research integrity [41].

A UK-based scientist in pharmacy practice was condemned to 3-month imprisonment against alteration of the preclinical trial data—procedures formulated in assistance of applications for performing the human trials. He worked on animal preclinical trials to assess the efficiency of recent treatment techniques alongside various bigger multinational drug companies, rather Aptuit has carried out the work. Eaton selectively reported fabricated data during his tenure at Aptuit to assess the working of analytical methods and the concentration of the drug in blood [42]. A General Practitioner from Downpatrick acted as Principal Investigator for an insomnia trial during 2007–2008 by Sanofi. He was jailed for falsifying drug trials in 2016 for conducting the trial deliberately breaching the protocol and conditions of good clinical practices. He is also the UK's first doctor for being condemned for falsifying data deliberately under the regulations of Medicines for Human Use (Clinical Trials) 2004 [43].

9.6 Importance of Data Integrity

Data integrity is an ethical and professional obligation that aims to provide definitive results toward the healthcare system and the governing authorities. This includes validation, accuracy, consistency, and quality of the data involved [44]. Data integrity is the cornerstone of scientific research, which showcases the research process commitment and trustworthiness [45]. Members of a scientific community need to function together, as a team, ensuring better research findings and exchange of research information to innovate and flourish, upholding professional and personal responsibility, acknowledging and respecting the intellectual contributions by the other members of the community [46].

Even if it is not digital, all the research data can be predisposed to misrepresentation and error. The electronic technologies and advancements can bring in some sources of technical error toward the communication, storage systems, or data analysis, making problematic data very difficult to separate from irrelevant information, due to which the methods of research cannot be strongly enacted, and even the asked questions may not be adequately explained [47]. Moreover, the researchers can get few benefits for structuring gathering data or research to favor a certain outcome, in cases such as the studies related to drugs funded by the pharmaceutical companies that nestle to profit across specific results. The researchers could have some "philosophical, political, or religious convictions" that can influence their work, which can also include the methods to gather and analyze data. Due to numerous data departure methods across the actualities, every individual included in the data collection, preservation, analysis, and dissemination has a discrete responsibility for safeguarding the integrity of the data [48].

Clinical trials that are conducted by the Contract Research Organizations (CRO) complete up to 30% more rapidly than those trials managed internally by the pharma companies. This helps in cost saving to a major extent, better utilization of clinical trials, and likely toward a faster market launch. With on-site monitoring, the overall cost of clinical trials can be compromised up to 25–30%, as monitoring is commonly the costliest facet of clinical trials. Risk-based monitoring, which has emerged over the last decade, is being encouraged by the regulatory authorities to reduce the monitoring expense [49].

Measures for ensuring data integrity are crucial to maintaining the research data in the long-term, including persistent questioning, in what way various organizations ensure the large datasets are to be stored in a relevant manner, indexed and referenced for future. Also, funding for effective data management should be made available to achieve long-term assessment and data conversation. Therefore, scientists and funding organizations or agencies should work on developing tools to manage the metadata, which could help the researchers annotate it and create required software. All these would help track individual pieces of data, which plays a major role for data-processing professionals to attain their scientific enterprise and be well recognized. Therefore, better education, training practices for the scientists pertaining to the data stewardship issues are essential. Training described above practices should include better analytics of data preservation and storage, organization, its annotation, and appreciation of the bioinformatic tools that are currently available [50].

9.7 How to Identify Research Misconduct?

The "Office of Research Integrity (ORI)" under the "Department of Health and Human Services" is the organization authorized to promote and foster research morale and integrity within "U.S. Public Health Service." It supervises the identification and inquiry of allegations related to research misconduct and finally makes resolutions on research misconduct findings accordingly. ORI also provides technical assistance if required to any of the Institutions which are responding to research misconduct allegations through its Rapid Response Technical Assistance Program. A finding of research misconduct under the federal policy requires whether the misconduct be committed knowingly or intentionally or recklessly; a notable departure from the applicable research community's acquired practices happened, and the allegation of research misconduct is proven by a superiority of evidence. All of these three elements should be presented for a finding of research misconduct through a full-fledged investigation [51].

9.7.1 Software for Data Verifiability

Plagiarism softwares are the critical components in ensuring a scientific research work's quality and data verifiability. Plagiarism detection softwares enable the research personnel to systematically detect and prevent plagiarism, which can reduce the incidence of research misconduct to some extent. This software assesses the similarity of content in the papers with published literature and other information types, comparing the author's text against the citations and abstracts in "PubMed/MEDLINE" with millions of Journal publications, books, and chapters from the leading publishers which may include "Elsevier, Lippincott, Sage, Springer, Ovid and Wiley Blackwell," and many others including conference proceedings and varied databases such as "EBSCOHost, Gale InfoTrac, and ProQuest." Additionally, the software detecting plagiarism also searches the internet for any similar content. A leading software program, 'iThenticate,' has its own web crawler that indexes more than "10 million web pages daily" (iThenticate, 2018). All types of documents, whether it is a manuscript, written assignment for courses, grants, theses and dissertations, other scholarly projects, or other types of reports, can be checked with the plagiarism detection software. "Turnitin," a leading product designed to check the originality of student research papers, was particularly made for classroom use and student work review. It can also be incorporated with the other learning management systems for students to review their papers before submitting them and teachers then to assess those papers during review [52].

9.7.2 Internal Audits (Preclinical and Clinical Research)

Internal audit is defined as an independent and systematic evaluation of the activities and documents related to trial in determining the conduct of trial-related activities evaluation, and the data records, analysis, and accuracy notified in accordance to the protocol, sponsor's Standard Operating Procedures (SOPs), practices and the regulatory requirements applicable. Auditing is a quality assurance function, evaluating the research work's compliance to recognize the standards, i.e., "International Council on Harmonization, FDA's Code of Federal Regulations, International Standards Organization and Standard Operating Procedures" [53].

9.7.3 Electronic Health Record (EHR)

Electronic health records (EHR) are being implemented successfully, where there has been a steeper advance in secondary HER use, particularly for research. EHR is being redesigned gradually to facilitate future research, and the major barriers toward EHR are adoption costs, acquisition, and maintenance. They provide opportunities for enhancing patient care, embedding the measures of performance in clinical practice, and improving the recognition and enrolment of patients and healthcare providers who are eligible for clinical research. EHRs on a larger scale can aid in the assessment of the new therapies or innovations in the healthcare delivery that can follow the enhanced outcomes or healthcare savings. EHRs can be potentially used in assessing study feasibility, streamline data collection, facilitate patient recruitment, conduct EHR-based observational solely, or comparative effectiveness studies or post-marketing randomized registry studies. The sustainability of using EHRs toward the clinical trials registration is directly dependent on the regulative acceptance of the practices and approach [54].

9.8 How to Prevent Data Misconduct?

Certain guidelines and measures should be adopted and adhered to prevent data misconduct as outlined below.

9.8.1 Guidelines and Measures at the Preclinical Level

9.8.1.1 Universal Code of Ethics for Scientists

The scientists' universal code of ethics is a public declaration of the responsibilities and values to be practiced by scientists. For instance, the universal ethical code of the UK has three main aims: (1) Encouraging ethical research, (2) facilitating scientists to think about the impacts and implications of their work, and (3) assisting the communication between the public and scientists on some of the challenging and complicated issues. Since this code is optional, the Institutions or scientists are instead encouraged to understand and think about how these guidelines can be related to their work [55].

The basic universal code of ethics is the bedrock of science's integrity and credibility, which are referred to as the representatives of all scientific disciplines. Compliance with these principles and values is required by all the scientists and Institutions where the scientific research is being conducted.

A few of the core principles of this Universal ethical code include:

1. **Diligence**—to present the objectives of conducting and intending research, presenting the research methods and procedures, interpreting the findings, information disclosure about possible threats, and potential applications and advantages anticipated in an intentional manner.
2. **Impartiality**—in the approach of the presenting or problem and in sharing the scientific basis and knowledge with the other people.
3. **Courage**—to challenge the views that contradict the scientific practices and knowledge that breach the fundamentals of scientific authenticity.

4. **Objectivity**—to solely interpret and conclude depending on the facts that have acceptable data and reasoning which can be subjected to verification, if required.
5. **Trustworthiness**—to conduct and present research, a condemning approach to the results, apprehension with details and diligence to collect, record, and store the data.
6. **Resistance**—toward any attempts that can exert external influence on the research conducted
7. **Openness**—Regarding the researcher's own scientific work during the discussions or meetings with the fellow scientists, which contributes to the development of knowledge by research findings publication and knowledge sharing with the community.
8. **Transparency**—during the collection, the analysis, and the data interpretation, is decided by the empirical data storage properly and available through the publications.
9. **Concern**—for the future generation of scientists that can be demonstrated by instructing the good ethical standards and norms to the students and the other subordinates involved
10. **Responsibility**—with regard to the participants (subjects) involved in research and the objects that include the cultural and environmental property.
11. **Reliability**—to acknowledge the fellow researchers' scientific achievements by providing adequate referencing to the sources and trustworthy recognition of the other scientist's contributions.

The universities, institutes, or other entities involved in research must be obliged to ensure that the employees of their respective organizations comply with the basic principles and ethics. Those Institutions are also expected to introduce and apply the explicit principles of good scientific practices and promote sensitivity toward ethical issues among their organizations [56]. Most of the countries have their own clinical research regulating authorities, e.g., Food and Drug Administration (FDA) for the United States Health Science Authority (HSA) for Singapore, Central Drug Standards Control Organization (CDSCO) for India, State Food and Drug Administration (SFDA), and Medicines and Healthcare Regulatory Agency (MHRA), etc.

9.8.1.2 Regulations and Measures to Prevent Data Misconduct

The role of Institutional Review Boards (IRBs) or Institutional Ethical Committees (IECs) should be strengthened to safeguard the interests of persons participating or conducting research [57]. There should be some internal regulatory and review procedures to monitor the ongoing studies' ethically acceptable and quality control characteristics. The regulations that are already in existence must be streamlined and made much efficient, ensuring that all the organizations or institutes, whoever associated with clinical research, should have clear policies and procedures for operating and approaching misconduct and fraud in research [58].

The division of roles for dealing with research misconduct allegations differs from one country to the other. The three generic ways for handling the misconduct cases, in general, are:

1. **Ad-hoc committees**—Generally consist of distinguished individuals, established for dealing with specific cases, preferably under the patronage of ethics committees that are already existing as university-based. The major advantage of this approach is the ready existence of ethics committees at various Institutions, as they are chiefly associated with life sciences and handling matters related to human experimental patients and subjects. It is difficult to ascertain if these committees can address all the research misconduct cases while these are very vital and essential. Extension of ethics committee directives to handle research misconduct cases must be seconded by cautious analysis and alterations of already existing procedures and rules if required.
2. **Standing committees**—Constitutes of entities or units (officers, committees, or offices) and procedures corresponding, at the institution level (e.g., bigger laboratory/university) where the misconduct happens in research Institutions. These standing committees can be answerable for accepting allegations, undertaking them (including conduct and necessary investigations), and proposing the outcomes. These entities are generally not autonomous, and there is an interaction measure with government-regulated central national bodies or authorities.
3. "**One or more dedicated committee(s)**"—Selected by the countries where the scientific communities in their regions are small, as it could be difficult for establishing impartial scientist committees, free of conflicts of interest personally at the national level. In such instances, to represent a greater spectrum of applicable expertise, "members of the permanent national committees" can be selected [59].

9.8.1.3 Audit of Data Values

Audit of data compares the contents of the study database to a local document source and noting the irregularities and disparities in the discrete data elements. The available document source could be the clinical records on paper, i.e., medical, pharmacy records, and electronic laboratory reports. Audit findings are expected to be documented on a well-structured audit form paper and entered into the Excel spreadsheets for further analysis. The audit variables could include those that are most relevant to the suggested consortium studies, for example, patient demographic data, risk factors, anthropometric measurements, etc., and all dates associated with each measurement. Audit of data functions as a beneficial control measure for data quality to the data coordinating center (DCC) as well as the participating sites, which allows the DCC for identifying and resolving the weaknesses in the data submitted, thereby preventing incorrect data from affecting the results of the study [60].

9.8.1.4 Good Laboratory Practices for Data Integrity

The Department of the Interior (DOI), USA defines Scientific integrity as the state or condition that applies to a person who adheres to the appropriate scientific community's acceptable standards, practices, and professional values [61]. Adhering to the acceptable standards is suggestive of ensuring clarity, fairness, utility, and authenticity of scholastic and scientific assessments that help in preventing scientific misconduct, licensing, outside interference, and adequate assurance of information and procedural security [62].

GLP was first introduced in the year 1972 in Denmark and New Zealand, and subsequently within the USA during the year 1978 after the scandal of Industrial BioTest Labs, which was then succeeded by the "Organization for Economic Co-operation and Development (OECD) Principles of GLP" in the year 1992—setting up OECD aided in propagating GLP to a large number of countries. Good Laboratory Practices (GLPs) are the formal regulations designed by the "U.S Food and Drug Administration (FDA)" in the year 1978. An "Expert Group on GLP" set up during 1978 built the first "Organisation for Economic Co-operation and Development (OECD) Principles of Good Laboratory Practice" for a special program on controlling the use of chemicals [63]. The GLP regulations put together by the US FDA in the year 1976 were undertaken as "international standards" toward the nonclinical laboratory-based studies that are published. Eventually, other countries too started making GLP regulations in their home countries after the USA [64].

Good Laboratory Practices are defined as the principles that provide a framework for planning, performing, recording, monitoring, reporting, and archiving laboratory studies. They offer a set of guidelines that govern the organization, procedures, processes, and conditions under which laboratory studies are conducted and executed, providing an assurance to the regulatory authorities regarding the data submitted, which will be an accurate reflection of the study results [65].

The Good Laboratory Practices (GLP) are centered around four major principles required for achieving good quality data. These also serve as essential functions in accordance to perform and monitor the safety studies. They include:

1. **Management**—has the overall responsibility to implement good organization and science within the Institutions
2. **Quality Assurance**—for assuring the management regarding personnel, facilities, records and practices are strict as per the regulations for maintaining the blueprints of the studies, inspecting every nonclinical study at regular timeframes to make sure about the compliance and reporting the results to management and the study director for reviewing the report finally.
3. **Study Director**—as a unique source of control for the study who must assure that the study protocol is acceptable and followed up accordingly, making sure that entire experimental data is adequately recorded and good GLPs are properly followed, and all the raw data, protocols, documentation, final reports, and specimens are registered effectively.
4. **The National Compliance Monitoring Authority**—an established body within a member country that should be responsible for keeping track of the good laboratory practice receptivity amongst the test facilities of its various areas and discharging other similar purposes associated with good laboratory practices determined nationwide [66].

The major concerns of GLPs for effective implementation are:

Data Records System (DRS) The raw electronic information providing the probability of conducting a complete audit trail can show modifications to the data without concealing the actual data. Associating all data changes by making those changes to the persons through timed and dated (electronic) signatures is required, and retention of the long-term data could be tough if the software and hardware associated with the data are quickly changing. The procedures should be documented well, and the verification of its integrity must be done, wherever the system obsoleteness poses a requirement for transferring the raw electronic data between the two different systems. The raw data should be transferred to the other medium where the migration is not practical, which is subsequently verified as an exact copy earlier to demolition the original electronic records, if any [67].

'Standard Operating Procedures (SOPs)' SOPs are the "written procedures" that are designed for a laboratory program, which are the "approved protocols" indicating the objectives and methods of a test/study. SOPs are intended toward ensuring the integrity and quality of data that is produced by the test facility. SOPs define the ways for carrying out activities specific to the protocols and are frequently written as a sequential listing of the action moves. They also explain the process and procedures for better working principles like calibration, maintenance, general inspection, and testing, actions that need to be taken in cases of failure of equipment, defining the raw data, reporting, keeping the records, data recovery, and storage. Every other test facility area or unit is recommended to possess one currently available manual of Standard Operating Procedures at least that is relevant to the activities which are being conducted therein to assure good clinical practices. Some special Standard Operating Procedures (SOPs) are laid down for the preparation, approval, and control of Standard Operating Procedures (SOPs), together called SOPs of SOPs. These SOPs of SOPs are applicable to prepare and implement all Standard Operating Procedures. Controlled Documents in SOPs constitute copies of mastered documents, distributed in the respective departments, which are stamped as Controlled Copy in Green Colour at the bottom right corner on each page. Uncontrolled documents are distributed to regulatory agencies, customers, or other persons if required, stamped in red ink made from master copies/ control copies of filled documents [68].

Peer Review Reviewing the study-specified or non-study-specific data will support recognizing the corresponding findings, which assist in interpreting and influencing the earlier identified microscopic findings [69].

Equipment The equipment that includes the certified computerized systems used for the "generation, storage, data recovery, and controlling the environmental factors" that are relevant and appropriate to the study must be located suitable and must be designed appropriately with an adequate capacity [70].

Records of Chemicals Used Chemicals or reagents of the lab should be labeled properly and appropriately to indicate the compound's identity source concentration and stability. A user must make an entry whenever he/she uses it in a specific log sheet.

It should also include the date of preparation, specific storage instructions, and the earliest expiration date [70]. The specific amount used/spent on chemicals should be entered as well as the remaining balance along with the user signature with date. This activity would help maintain the chemical usage record, which is essential for the tracking of the experiments as well as accountability of the chemicals to avoid deficits in usage and unnecessary purchase. Quality assurance personnel must ensure this practice and proper compliance by the users on a monthly or quarterly basis.

GLP always aims to reduce the mistake occurrences via extensive and more specific labeling prerequisites. As the principles of Good Laboratory Practice (GLP) are developed to promote the validity and quality of test data can be applied for determining the chemicals and the other chemical product's safety. These GLPs also protect the researcher from unfounded allegations that could even benefit the institution or the laboratory. The Food and Drug Administration (FDA) is the organization for validation of the study to report the reflections of conduct of the study accurately, while the GLP regulations, that are framed to promulgate the standards of the laboratory. Eventually, every study is generally compared to the FDA's expectations that progress over time within the regulatory framework. The Quality control and the GLP rules are the process that all the laboratories try to opt for, which is the way forward for the "evidence-based laboratory results" based on trustworthy procedure [71].

9.8.1.5 Preclinical Guidelines (OECDs)

"Organisation for Economic Co-operation and Development (OECD)" is an internationally reputed agency working for framing better policies toward the better and finer lives. Their objective is to outline the policies fostering "prosperity, opportunity, equality, and wellbeing for all." OECD works "together with the governments, policymakers, and citizens to establish evidence-based international standards and find solutions that range around social, economic, and environmental challenges." The OECD dispenses a distinctive knowledge and forum hub toward analyzing data, experiencing exchange, sharing best practices, and guiding international standard-setting and public policies. Mutual Acceptance of Data (MAD) system, a multilateral agreement developed by the OECD, allows countries to participate in public policies and include non-members for sharing their results of various nonclinical investigations done on the chemicals using OECD methods and principles [72].

9.8.1.6 Checklist for Preclinical Studies for Data Verifiability

Data verifiability and irreproducibility of preclinical scientific research are the core principles for ensuring the quality and transparency of research and reporting. Hence, it is suggested for the authors to complete a checklist at the time of the manuscript submission. Data auditing within the preclinical settings and studies is the essential strategy that is extensively used as a significant way forward in identifying errors, monitoring operations of the study, and ensuring superior-quality data. The reliability of quality data assessment can be undermined due to the absence of a precise definition of data quality and error measuring methods [73].

9.8.1.7 Journal Policies

Committee on Publication Ethics (COPE) is a global organization committed to aiding and training the publishers, editors, and the personnel engaged in maintaining the publication ethics with the aim of passing on the publishing culture where ethical procedures and practices turn out to be a normal routine. The approach of COPE is firmly along the direction of influence by educating, providing resources and support to the members, along with the professional debate strengthening the wider community. The journal's policies are framed to maintain the research integrity and the quality published in their journals. This holds the responsibility for the authenticity of scientific observations or findings, precision of statements of fact, scientific expression or other opinions, and any other published material in the journal lies solely with the article author(s). The journal policies are classified as (1). Editorial and Publishing policies, and (2). Peer-review policies. Editorial and publishing policies are related to submitting the manuscript, transferring the manuscript rights from the authors to the journal, responsibilities of the author, and data integrity maintenance. Peer reviewing policies mainly run around the manuscript's peer review process from the initial submission to the final decision on the document. These policies are laid to showcase the quality and transparency of the journal and its procedures [74].

9.8.1.8 Publication Ethics

Scientific research includes a lot of coordinated steps and processes, including the appropriate study design and execution, data collection, processing and analysis, and finally the publication. Every researcher should be aware of the ethical code of conduct that binds them and regulates them. Good ethical standards for the publication of research work exist to ensure superior-quality scientific publications and trust among the public in the scientific findings. The people who conducted the research receive credit for their ideas. An international publisher and editor's forum of peer-reviewed journals, the Committee on Publication Ethics (COPE) provides the "best practice guidelines" and "code of conduct," which defines the publication ethics and advises editors regarding the handling cases of research and publication misconduct. The authors should be aware of publication ethics that can help them consciously avoid scientific misconduct and perform honest and acceptable ethical research [75].

9.8.1.9 Authorship Consent Form

The authors of a manuscript transfers the rights to the publishing company or agency by giving their consent through a form called an Authorship consent form. This also includes the publication rights of nonexclusive, and the authors must assure about the originality of their contribution. All the authors sign the consent form as an acceptance of the responsibility to release the material on behalf of them and publication rights transfer covering the nonexclusive part of the rights for reproducing alongside the research article distribution. The protocols and scientific manuscripts must be seconded by a completed author consent form or cover letter during submission, that include the details such as:

1. A complete affirmation to the editor or relevant authoritative person regarding all the submissions and previous reports, if any.
2. An affirmation on authorship, which can require a letter of submission including a statement about the manuscript, was read and accepted by each author of the article, making sure all the requirements for authorship are clearly understood.
3. An affirmation pertaining to financial or other activities and associations that can direct toward a conflict of interest, when such details are not mentioned within the manuscript or in an authors' form.
4. The author's contact information serves as an interface with the other authors regarding final approval or revision of the proofs when that particular information is not included in the manuscript.

The author consent form must also notify the journal editors if there are any concerns or issues raised or put up (e.g., the Institutional regulatory bodies) concerning the research conduct or any action required [76].

9.8.2 Guidelines and Measures at the Clinical Level

9.8.2.1 Clinical Guidelines: ICH

The "International Council for Harmonisation (ICH) of technical requirements for pharmaceuticals for human use (ICH)" is a global organization, which is unique at its work to bring the regulatory authorities and pharmaceutical industries together for discussing the technical and scientific aspects of registering a drug. It was set up in the year 1990, had its evolution progressively in response to the growing global overlook of drug development. Its goal is to attain harmonization to more considerable extent globally for ensuring effective, safe, and superior-quality medicines being registered and developed in a much resourceful manner. The ICH Guidelines development attains this harmonization through a scientific consensus process with industry and regulatory experts working alongside.

The topics recognized for "harmonization" by the "ICH Steering Committee" are picked out from the quality, safety, multidisciplinary, and efficacy affairs. Quality topics include pharmaceutical and chemical quality assurance (Impurity Testing, Stability Testing, etc.). Effectiveness topics include those associated with the human subject clinical studies (Good Clinical Practices, Dose-Response Studies, etc). Topics of safety include those related to "in vivo and in vitro preclinical studies (Genotoxicity Testing, Carcinogenicity Testing," etc. Interdisciplinary areas or topics include e cross-cutting topics that do not fit individually into any of the above categories.

The ICH guidelines are classified as follows:

Carcinogenicity studies (S1A-S1C):

S1A Guidelines on the need for pharmaceuticals' carcinogenicity studies, guiding studies pertaining to carcinogenicity performed for any pharmaceutical industry.

S1B Testing for pharmaceutical carcinogenicity, providing instructions regarding the need to carry out carcinogenicity studies on both rats and mice.

S1C(R2) Dose selection for pharmaceutical carcinogenicity studies, addressing criteria for selecting high dose to be used in carcinogenicity studies

S2—Genotoxicity:

S2(R1) Guidance on Genotoxicity testing and interpretation of data for the pharmaceuticals intended for human use

S2B A standard battery for Genotoxicity testing for pharmaceuticals, addressing two fundamental areas pertaining to genotoxicity testing: identification and registration of a standard set of assays

S3A-S3B toxicokinetics and pharmacokinetics:

S3A Guidance on Toxicokinetics: systemic exposure assessment in the toxicity studies, giving instructions on developing test strategies in toxicokinetics

S3B Pharmacokinetics: Guidance for repeated dose tissue distribution studies

S4 Chronic toxicity duration testing in animals, rodent and non-rodent toxicity testing

S5 Toxicity detection toward reproduction for medicinal products and toxicity to male fertility

S6 Evaluating the preclinical safety of biotechnology-derived pharmaceuticals, where the preclinical safety evaluation of primary goals is to identify the initial safe and subsequent dose in humans and potential target organs for toxicity and for the study of whether such toxicity is reversible and safety parameters for clinical monitoring.

S7A Safety pharmacological studies for human pharmaceuticals, generated toward protecting participants and patients of clinical trials who receive marketed products from the pharmaceutical's potential adverse effects.

S7B Nonclinical evaluation of the potential by human pharmaceuticals for the delayed ventricular repolarization (Q.T. interval prolongation)

S8 Immunotoxicity Studies for Human Pharmaceuticals, addressing the regulations and recommendations on immunosuppressant nonclinical testing.

S9 Anticancer Pharmaceuticals nonclinical evaluation, providing information for pharmaceuticals that are intended only to treat cancer in patients with advanced disease or later stage regardless of the administration route

S10 Photo safety evaluation of pharmaceuticals, addresses clinical formulation excipients for photodynamic therapy products and dermal applications.

S11 For safety nonclinical testing in support of pediatric medicines development recommend standards for the circumstances under which nonclinical juvenile testing of animals is considered informing

The ICH M3 (R2) guideline states that "conduct of any study related to juvenile animal toxicity must be taken into consideration when human safety and animal data are considered to be sufficient enough for supporting the pediatric studies" [77].

9.8.2.2 Clinical Trial Registry

Clinical Trials Registry by the government is the biggest registry, accepting trials from all over the world, taking steps to detect and avoid probable duplicates whenever identified, keeping only a single version of the trial data active. The clinical trial registration occurs prospectively, which is a scientific and ethical imperative phenomenon whose critical goal is to recognize all the ongoing or already conducted trials appropriate to a given topic. Duplicates of a trial can occur through purposeful or intentional registration of the trial by a person belonging to that trial or uncoordinated enrollment of trial by different people of the same trial. World Health Organization (WHO), through its Mexico statement, addressed the problem of duplicate trial registration, after which it called for "unambiguous identification" of every trial, directed toward the formation of the "International Clinical Trials Registry Platform (ICTRP)" by the WHO. WHO had also created the Universal Trial Number (UTN) scheme to facilitate the explicit recognition of trials by allotment of a distinctive number to that trial related to the trial for its lifetime. An explicit identification of trials essential to prevent double or triple counting of the evidence in systematic reviews and meta-analyses and ensure all the registry records that describe each relevant trial could be identified and retrieved. Hence, the explicit recognition of any trial is a major step to enhance systematic reviews' efficiency and effectiveness using information technology [78].

9.8.2.3 Checklist for Clinical Studies for Data Verifiability

Data verifiability and irreproducibility of clinical scientific research are the core principles for ensuring the quality and transparency of research and reporting. Hence, it is suggested for the authors to complete a checklist at the time of the manuscript submission. Data auditing within clinical settings and studies is the essential strategy that is extensively used as a major strategy in identifying errors, monitoring operations of the study, and ensuring superior-quality data. Nevertheless, the guidelines for clinical trials are not specific to the suggested frequency, nature, and timing of the data audits. The reliability of quality data assessment can be undermined due to the absence of a precise definition of data quality and error measuring methods [73].

9.9 Penalty for Data Fraud or Misconduct

The research institutions or organizations can penalize the researchers, those who are fond of having committed scientific misconduct, through requiring supervision of future research activities or terminating their employment depending on the act. The grantee of a research project should evaluate the impact of the research outcome on that person's ability to continue their work on that research project when the grantee institution or agency finds that person guilty of misconduct in research. "Office of Research Integrity (ORI)," an esteemed international organization, imposes penalties toward research misconduct, where the liability for the misconduct depends on the extremity of misconduct. The aspects that ORI can think about while picking up a penalty can comprise of the extent of misconduct or committed knowingly, intentionally, or carelessly, any notable influence on the records and subjects of the research, other institutions, researchers, or public well-being. "Office of Research Integrity (ORI)" can even enforce various penalties if the research misconduct is upheld, including Terminating or Suspending the research grant. Suspending or debarred from receiving federal funds in the future, or simply by correcting the research record or letters of reprimand. ORI will promptly refer the issue to an investigating body if it considers that the scientific misconduct might have been associated with criminal or civil fraud [79].

The regulations in India by University Grants Commission (UGC) for scientific misconduct are categorized based on the plagiarism of those scientific materials. Research publications' misconduct is considered a least serious offence when 10% of a manuscript is plagiarized, while the papers containing 60% or more plagiarized material can be considered the most serious offence. There are no penalties levied on the researchers whose papers have 10% or less plagiarized material. A student could be removed from their course, and a researcher would be required to retract their paper if that paper or material is found to be in the most serious plagiarism category. There are also other repercussions for the researchers as they cannot receive a pay raise for 2 years or will not be allowed to supervise a student's dissertation for 3 years [80]. A total of 106 papers problematic papers were retracted from "Council of Scientific and Industrial—Research Indian Institute of Toxicology Research (CSIR-IITR)" in 2019, which were found listed on the Pubpeer website for image manipulation and duplication

9.10 False Allegation of Research Misconduct

As the incidence of scientific misconduct is documented well, the issues about innocence and its establishment in the cases of false allegations are not addressed effectively. Hence, the investigators must be careful enough and need to assimilate the procedures to protect themselves in cases of untrue allegations. Essentiality for proving the innocence from the false allegations by the scientific community's people carries a more comprehensive range of responsibilities that can even exceed the normal legal assumptions. Researchers and Scientists across the world must be well prepared to safeguard their reputation and credibility by proper organization and maintenance of every single original file and the datasheet that is related to their grant proposals and publications, which they should be in a position to put forth all those documents to prove their transparency at any moment when such allegations and concerns are put up [81].

The government regulations for these allegations about the organizational procedures and policies involve two main phases, an inquiry and an investigation. A preliminary evaluation into the allegation with the other details for determining the adequate ground to investigate further into the allegations of misconduct comes under the inquiry phase. At the same time, the investigation involves formal examination and evaluation of relevant information for determining the occurrence of misconduct. The scientific research procedure can regularly fix the allegations or disagreements that may involve queries against the questionable research practices or scientific judgment can be regularly fixed by the procedure of the scientific research itself questionable research practices or scientific judgment. The proper management of misconduct allegations is long-standing, challenging, and even costly, which can divert faculty and administrative attention from other vital issues. Hence, the false allegations must be carefully dealt with and solved accordingly in a well-structured manner [82].

9.11 Future Directions and Clinical Implications

It is essential to have procedures in place for the early identification of patterns indicating data issues and concerns. The methods and protocols to ensure data quality in clinical trials that include data fraud identification and management must be progressed toward expansion and refinement if required. Central statistical monitoring techniques for ensuring the data integrity of clinical trials could be used heavily for suggesting remedial actions during the trial. Statistical assessments for the data quality can be proved useful during peer review, as journal editors can request access to the source data more often beyond which claims can be made. Open discussions among the researchers worldwide on the data integrity aspect of clinical research and their regular discussions will help reduce the incidence of data fraud.

9.12 Conclusion

Each country should have an official body that investigates and judges clinical or basic research fraud. All the organizations involved in the preclinical and clinical research must have concerning authorities functioning. To carry out transparent policies, strategies, and Standard Operating Procedures (SOPs), that can uplift the misconduct disclosures. Scientific fraud must be regarded as a serious issue without neglecting the actual causes. Transparent communications between the research groups on a crucial feature of clinical research besides discussing the already happening practices and projects can help reduce the fraud and misconduct incidence.

References

1. Godlee F, Smith J, Marcovitch H. Wakefield's article linking MMR vaccine and autism was fraudulent. BMJ. 2011;342:c7452.
2. Institute of Medicine, National Academy of Sciences, National Academy of Engineering. On being a scientist: a guide to responsible conduct in research. Washington, DC: National Academies Press; 2009.
3. Fanelli D. How many scientists fabricate and falsify research? A systematic review and meta-analysis of survey data. PLoS One. 2009;4:e5738.

4. Judson HF. The great betrayal: fraud in science. Orlando, FL: Harcourt; 2004.
5. Newton RR. The crime of claudius ptolemy. Baltimore, MD: Johns Hopkins University Press; 1977.
6. Galton D. Did Mendel falsify his data? QJM Int J Med. 2012;105:215–6.
7. Stroebe W, Postmes T, Spears R. Scientific misconduct and the myth of self-correction in science. Perspect Psychol Sci. 2012;7:670–88.
8. Retraction—Ileal-lymphoid-nodular hyperplasia, non-specific colitis, and pervasive developmental disorder in children. Lancet. 2010;375:445.
9. Ball P. Anti-vaccine movement could undermine efforts to end coronavirus pandemic, researchers warn. Nature. 2020;581:251.
10. Boetto E, Golinelli D, Carullo G, Fantini MP. Frauds in scientific research and how to possibly overcome them. J Med Ethics. 2020; https://doi.org/10.1136/medethics-2020-106639.
11. Miller DR. Retraction of articles written by Dr. Yoshitaka Fujii. Can J Anaesth. 2012;59:1081–8.
12. Neema PK. Dishonesty in medical research and publication and the remedial measures. Ann Card Anaesth. 2018;21:111–3.
13. Saikia P, Thakuria B. Retraction of papers authored by Yuhji Saitoh—beyond the Fujii phenomenon. Indian J Anaesth. 2019;63:571–84.
14. Bauchner H, Fontanarosa PB, Flanagin A, Thornton J. Scientific misconduct and medical journals. JAMA. 2018;320:1985–7.
15. Deshmukh MA, Dodamani AS, Khairnar MR, Naik RG. Research misconduct: a neglected plague. Indian J Public Health. 2017;61:33–6.
16. Zietman AL. Falsification, fabrication, and plagiarism: the unholy trinity of scientific writing. Int J Radiat Oncol Biol Phys. 2013;87:225–7.
17. Sarwar U, Nicolaou M. Fraud and deceit in medical research. J Res Med Sci. 2012;17:1077–81.
18. Singal J. Michael LaCour probably fabricated a document about research integrity. New York Magazine. 2015. Retrieved from: http://nymag.com/scienceofus/2015/06/lacour-probably-fabricated-an-integrity-document.html.
19. Kekre NS. Scientific misconduct—why we must be careful. Indian J Urol. 2012;28:247.
20. Habermann B, Broome M, Pryor ER, Ziner KW. Research coordinators' experiences with scientific misconduct and research integrity. Nurs Res. 2010;59:51–7.
21. Gupta A. Fraud and misconduct in clinical research: a concern. Perspect Clin Res. 2013;4:144–7.
22. Jump P. A star's collapse: Dutch begin documenting and trying to explain top psychologist's massive fraud. Inside Higher Ed. 2011. Retrieved from: https://www.insidehighered.com/news/2011/11/28/scholars-analyze-case-massive-research-fraud.
23. Berlinck RG. The academic plagiarism and its punishments—a review. Revista Brasileira de Farmacognosia. 2011;21:365–72.
24. Masic I. Plagiarism in scientific publishing. Acta Informatica Medica. 2012;20:208.
25. Reddy VS. Greetings from Davangere, Karnataka, India: searching versus researching. J Indian Soc Pedod Prev Dent. 2011;29:1.
26. Sharma BB, Singh V. Ethics in writing: learning to stay away from plagiarism and scientific misconduct. Lung India Off Organ Indian Chest Soc. 2011;28:148.
27. Rathod SD. Combating plagiarism: a shared responsibility. Indian J Med Ethics. 2010;7(3):173–5.
28. Rossner M, Yamada KM. What's in a picture? The temptation of image manipulation. J Cell Biol. 2004;166:11–5.
29. Frow EK. Drawing a line: setting guidelines for digital image processing in scientific journal articles. Soc Stud Sci. 2012;42:369–92.
30. Rossner M, O'Donnell R. The JCB will let your data shine in RGB. New York: Rockefeller University Press; 2004.
31. Angra A, Gardner SM. Reflecting on graphs: attributes of graph choice and construction practices in biology. CBE Life Sci Educ. 2017;16:ar53.
32. Simundic A-M. Bias in research. Biochemia Medica. 2013;23:12–5.

33. Jeffrey Brainard JY. What a massive database of retracted papers reveals about science publishing's 'death penalty'. Science Editing. Available at: https://www.sciencemag.org/news/2018/10/what-massive-database-retracted-papers-reveals-about-science-publishing-s-death-penalty. Accessed 28 Oct 2020.
34. Retractionwatch. Which countries have the most retractions, for which reasons? J Med Libr Asso. Available at: https://retractionwatch.com/2014/05/15/which-countries-have-the-most-retractions-for-which-reasons/. Accessed 28 Oct 2020.
35. Vuong QH, La V-P, Hồ MT, Vuong T-T, Ho M-T. Characteristics of retracted articles based on retraction data from online sources through February 2019. Sci Editing. 2020;7:34–44.
36. Amos KA. The ethics of scholarly publishing: exploring differences in plagiarism and duplicate publication across nations. J Med Libr Assoc JMLA. 2014;102:87.
37. Stretton S, Bramich NJ, Keys JR, Monk JA, Ely JA, Haley C, Woolley MJ, Woolley KL. Publication misconduct and plagiarism retractions: a systematic, retrospective study. Curr Med Res Opin. 2012;28:1575–83.
38. Patel M. Misconduct in clinical research in India: perception of clinical research professional in India. J Clin Res Bioeth. 2017;8:303.
39. Fang FC, Steen RG, Casadevall A. Misconduct accounts for the majority of retracted scientific publications. Proc Natl Acad Sci USA. 2012;109:17028–33.
40. Al-Marzouki S, Roberts I, Marshall T, Evans S. The effect of scientific misconduct on the results of clinical trials: a Delphi survey. Contemp Clin Trials. 2005;26:331–7.
41. Ankier S. Dishonesty, misconduct and fraud in clinical research: an international problem. J Int Med Res. 2002;30:357–65.
42. Benderly B. A prison sentence for altering data. Sci Careers. 2013.
43. Dyer C. GP accused of fraudulently conducting a clinical trial. BMJ (Online). 2016;352.
44. Macrina FL. Methods, manners, and the responsible conduct of research. Washington, DC: ASM Press; 2005.
45. Mabrouk PA. The ethical chemist: professionalism and ethics in science (Jeffrey Kovac). ACS; 2004.
46. N.R. Council. US National Academy of Sciences. Confronting Natural Disasters: US National Academy of Engineering; 1987.
47. Davies EB. Science in the looking glass: what do scientists really know? Oxford University Press on Demand; 2003.
48. Krimsky S. Publication bias, data ownership and the funding effect in science: threats to the integrity of biomedical research. In: Rescuing science from politics: regulation and the distortion of scientific research. 2006. p. 61–85.
49. Getz KA. Uncovering the drivers of R&D costs. In: 2015 presentation citing data from the Tufts Center for the Study of Drug Development. Accessible at: http://www.clinicalleader.com/doc/the-need-for-speed-in-study-startup-0001.
50. Gov.UK. Universal ethical code for scientists. Available at: https://www.gov.uk/government/publications/universal-ethical-code-for-scientists. Accessed 21 Oct 2020.
51. Handling misconduct—inquiry & investigation issues. Office of Research Integrity. Retrieved from: https://ori.hhs.gov/content/ori-responses-issues. Accessed 29 Nov 2020.
52. Baždarić K. Plagiarism detection–quality management tool for all scientific journals. Croat Med J. 2012;53:1–3.
53. Park S, Nam CM, Park S, Noh YH, Ahn CR, Yu WS, Kim BK, Kim SM, Kim JS, Rha SY. 'Screening audit' as a quality assurance tool in good clinical practice compliant research environments. BMC Med Ethics. 2018;19:30.
54. Cowie MR, Blomster JI, Curtis LH, Duclaux S, Ford I, Fritz F, Goldman S, Janmohamed S, Kreuzer J, Leenay M. Electronic health records to facilitate clinical research. Clin Res Cardiol. 2017;106:1–9.
55. Ensuring data integrity. Nat Neurosci. 2009;12:1205.
56. Jones NL. A code of ethics for the life sciences. Sci Eng Ethics. 2007;13:25–43.
57. Cressey D. British science needs integrity overhaul. 2012. See http://www.nature.com/news/britishscience-needs-integrity-overhaul-1.9803. Last checked 2 July 2013.

58. Wilmshurst P. Dishonesty in medical research. Med Leg J. 2007;75:3–12.
59. Duda SN, Shepherd BE, Gadd CS, Masys DR, McGowan CC. Measuring the quality of observational study data in an international HIV research network. PLoS One. 2012;7:e33908.
60. Börner K. Organization for Economic Co-operation and Development: Global Science Forum workshop on science of science policy: developing our understanding of public investments in science. 2006
61. U.S. Department of Health and Human Services Office of Research Integrity. Case summaries. 2017. Available at: https://ori.hhs.gov/case_summary. Accessed 23 Oct 2020
62. Kretser A, Murphy D, Bertuzzi S, Abraham T, Allison DB, Boor KJ, Dwyer J, Grantham A, Harris LJ, Hollander R, Jacobs-Young C, Rovito S, Vafiadis D, Woteki C, Wyndham J, Yada R. Scientific integrity principles and best practices: recommendations from a Scientific Integrity Consortium. Sci Eng Ethics. 2019;25:327–55.
63. Becker RA, Janus ER, White RD, Kruszewski FH, Brackett RE. Good laboratory practices and safety assessments. Environ Health Perspect. 2009;117:A482-3. Author reply A483-4
64. Gladney L, Izabella O, Endia F. Good laboratory practices. 2009.
65. Zgheib N, Branch R, Buch S. Good clinical practice and good laboratory practice, Clinical and translational science. Elsevier; 2009, p. 345–60.
66. Salminen WF, Fowler JM, Greenhaw J. Nonclinical study contracting and monitoring: a practical guide. Academic; 2012.
67. Jean C. GLP: Good laboratory practice for field and research, ALS; 2007.
68. Anderson MA. GLP quality audit manual. Interpharm; 2000.
69. Robinson K. GLPs and the importance of standard operating procedures. Biopharm Int. 2003;16:38–47.
70. Klimisch HJ, Andreae M, Tillmann U. A systematic approach for evaluating the quality of experimental toxicological and ecotoxicological data. Regul Toxicol Pharmacol. 1997;25:1–5.
71. COP. Ethics, Core practices. 2017.
72. van Valkenhoef G, Loane RF, Zarin DA. Previously unidentified duplicate registrations of clinical trials: an exploratory analysis of registry data worldwide. Syst Rev. 2016;5:116.
73. Sengupta S, Honavar SG. Publication ethics. Indian J Ophthalmol. 2017;65:429–32.
74. Branch SK. Guidelines from the international conference on harmonisation (ICH). J Pharm Biomed Anal. 2005;38:798–805.
75. Sending the manuscript to the journal. International Committee of Medical Journal Editors (ICMJE). Retrieved from: http://www.icmje.org/recommendations/browse/manuscript-preparation/sending-the-submission.html. Accessed 28 Nov 2020.
76. Ginger C. Good laboratory practice CFR 21 Part 58. A review for OCRA US RAC Study Group, September 2005.
77. Organisation for Economic Co-operation, and Development. OECD recommendation on the governance of clinical trials. 2012.
78. Krishnankutty B, Bellary S, Kumar NB, Moodahadu LS. Data management in clinical research: an overview. Indian J Pharmacol. 2012;44:168–72.
79. Dal-Ré R, Bouter LM, Cuijpers P, Gluud C, Holm S. Should research misconduct be criminalized? Res Ethics. 2020;16:1–12.
80. Sabir H, Kumbhare S, Parate A, Kumar R, Das S. Scientific misconduct: a perspective from India. Med Health Care Philos. 2015;18:177–84.
81. Goldenring JR. Perspective: Innocence and due diligence: managing unfounded allegations of scientific misconduct. Acad Med. 2010;85:527–30.
82. National Academy of Sciences (US), National Academy of Engineering (US) and Institute of Medicine (US) Panel on Scientific Responsibility and the Conduct of Research. Responsible science: ensuring the integrity of the research process, vol II. National Academy Press; 1992.

The Role of Document Control and Archiving Records in Laboratory Management

10

Navneet Kaur, Prashant Verma, Bhavya Mody, Neeru Malik, Gurmeet Singh, and Chirayu Padhiar

10.1 Introduction: Document Control and Archiving

A document control system is one of the most critical tools for ensuring compliance in highly regulated laboratories or industries. Document control system is an integral part of the quality management system and enables the laboratory to be in compliance with relevant regulatory and accreditation requirements, whether it is in drug discovery, drug manufacturing, clinical research, hospitals, or clinical laboratories. Document control is one of the key requirements of ISO standards. It is good to remember that there are no consequences of doing too much but of doing too little. The management and control of records are one of the key features of the Quality management system in Good Laboratory Practices (GLP) facilities. Proper rules, regulations and guidelines, ethical code of conduct need to be followed by various personnel in the GLP system. Well-documented guidelines act as a source of guidance for an insider as well as an outsider in the laboratory. For the preparation and generation of documents, a proper systematic approach needs to be

N. Kaur · G. Singh
Department of Physical Education, Panjab University, Chandigarh, India

P. Verma
Interdisciplinary Centre for Swami Vivekananda Studies, Panjab University, Chandigarh, India

B. Mody
Kasturba Medical College, Manipal Academy of Higher Education, Manipal, Karnataka, India

N. Malik
Dev Samaj College of Education, Sector, 36-B, Chandigarh, India

C. Padhiar (✉)
LifeCell International Pvt. Ltd., Chennai, Tamil Nadu, India
e-mail: drchirayu.p@lifecell.in

A. Anand (ed.), *Quality Assurance Implementation in Research Labs*,
https://doi.org/10.1007/978-981-16-3074-3_10

followed for authenticated data generation like DRS, SOPs, log sheets, and master schedule, etc. Document control is imperative for the smooth conduct of experiments and retention of records in the GLP facilities. India has emphasized the need and importance of coding in its New Education Policy (NEP) 2020. In the previous years, the Government of India has changed its policies, and funding/approval agencies are taking strict actions against the companies/labs that have a lack of transparency in their documentation work. In order to avoid this situation and to make the defense strong, it becomes all the more important to follow GDP (Good Documentation Practices). GDP ensures an auditable account of the work performed and data integrity, thus ensuring compliance to national and international regulatory requirements. GDP individually and collectively must ensure **documentation** (electronic or paper), that is secure, attributable, legible, traceable, permanent, correctly recorded, original, and accurate.

Document control procedure provides a systemic process to prepare, review, approve, and publish a document or record. In addition, it should define the process for any updation or amendments and to archive the document when it is made obsolete. A document is not the same as a record. A document is written in the present and is forward-looking, whereas a record is related to the past and is back traceable. Both documents and records play important roles in GLP systems [1]. A document provides a controlled communication system within the organization. One might forget/misinterpret verbal instructions but written instructions mentioned in the document assist in better management of the Quality System.

Apart from document control, archival is also an important aspect of Good Documentation Practices. Archiving practices secure not only the data but also create space for a better working environment. Archiving involves storing the data that is not being used currently but may be required in the future.

According to the World Health Organization (WHO), document hierarchy follows the policies, processes, and procedures in the written form as shown in Fig. 10.1 [1].

1. **Policy:**

   The Policy provides the overall outline and direction on "what needs to be done." It includes the aim, objectives, and overview given by the top management. For example, a policy statement regarding "leave from work" should include a policy statement headline, along with the reason and the scope of its implementation, e.g., for permanent employees, contract employees, etc. [1]
2. **Process:**

   The Process is based on the principle of input and output. It gives the direction of flow regarding "how it happens," which involves steps for Quality management [1].
3. **Procedures:**

   Procedures involve detailed instructions of every step of performing a task in the laboratory [1, 2]. Procedures give the direction or instructions for "how to do" the particular task. The stepwise instructions need to be followed by the staff members of GLP facilities in a diligent way for quality data generation.

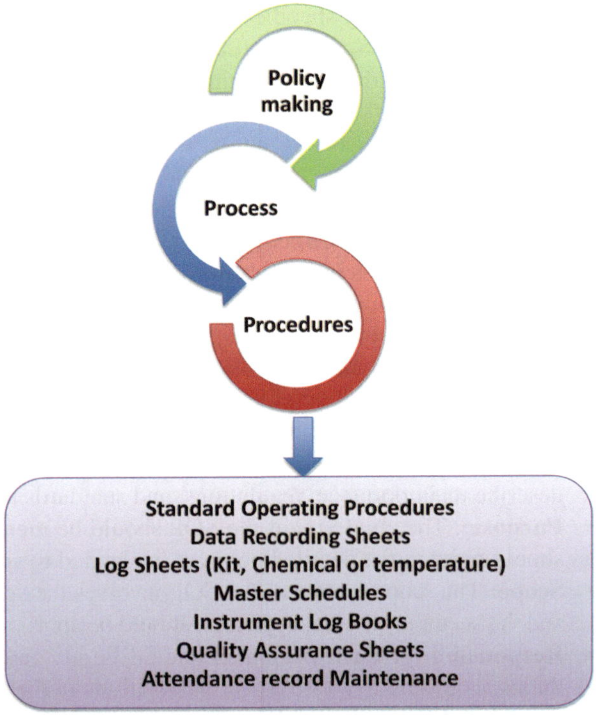

Fig. 10.1 The flow of Document control [1]

According to 21 CFR 820, every controlled document must clearly state [3]:

(a) Who generated the document?
(b) Who evaluated or validated the document and data?
(c) Who and when sanctioned the document?
(d) What is the status of the documents (Original, amended, revised, revalidated, awaiting approval)?
(e) The revision number of the Document.
(f) Approval (registered copy or official printout with signatures).

10.2 Standard Operating Procedure [4]

10.2.1 Overview

An SOP is the documented procedure of describing any operation. It provides the step-by-step details to deal with any task or experiment accurately and precisely. An SOP is usually designed for a specific task (e.g., In the management of hospital). SOPs can be universal. An example is "laboratory safety precautions" which remains the same irrespective of which laboratory is conducting the test. Other

SOPs can be laboratory specific or task specific. For example, estimation of protein content in the blood. Some SOPs can also be condition specific—for example, cryopreservation of blood in a liquid nitrogen Dewar.

10.2.2 SOP Content

An SOP should be a well-focused and concise document. For example, an SOP on the estimation of protein by Bradford method should include only that particular procedure. It is irrelevant to include details about protein estimation by the Lowri method or electrophoresis.

An SOP should contain the following elements:

- **Introduction:** Background information on the scope of work being undertaken should be mentioned. For example, an SOP on good laboratory practices should describe its importance, regulations, and standards that need to be adhered to etc.
- **Purpose:**. The chief aim of the SOP should be mentioned briefly and clearly. It should point to the detailed policy it is planned to support.
- **Scope:** The scope or area of the SOP involves the specific activities that it covers and the scenario where it applies. It should be appropriately mentioned in the SOP.
- **Responsibility:** Each personnel should be allocated their responsibilities and duties according to their respective positions in the Laboratory.
- **Associated Records and Forms**: Any related SOPs, standardized forms, benchmarks, and other source documents must be enlisted. Moreover, any related record-keeping document should also be mentioned. Provide examples of forms to be utilized and mention how it needs to be accomplished.
- **Materials Required:** Describe the specific equipment, consumables or reagents that are required.
- **Procedure:** Clear, accurate, and stepwise instructions for procedures need to be followed. Furthermore**,** use illustrations, presentations, and images wherever required.
- **Distribution:** Maintain or register the record of the distribution of the SOP along with its revisions, updates, or amendments. Moreover, SOPs that are older and suspended versions need to be withdrawn.
- **Risk Assessment:** If there is any risk involved in a particular test or experiment, the safety provisions should be clearly mentioned to alleviate it.
- **Training:** Provide details regarding any type of training, if required.

10.2.3 How Should SOPs Be Used?

For the SOP to be used in a particular work area(s), it must be readily accessible there. The concerned personnel must also know the exact location of the document. Moreover, the supervisor must ensure that new appointees are trained to follow the SOPs related to their assigned duties.

STANDARD OPERATING PROCEDURE

Institute logo/Name

<table>
<tr><td colspan="6">Title: ARCHIVING</td></tr>
<tr><td>SOP No.
AB12-YZ-34</td><td>Edition No.
01</td><td colspan="2">Effective Date</td><td>Review Date</td><td rowspan="2">Document Controller
(Signature/Stamp)</td></tr>
<tr><td>Copy No.1</td><td colspan="2">Date of Issue</td><td colspan="2">Location (Unit/Division)</td></tr>
</table>

Fig. 10.2 Template to design an SOP

10.2.4 Designing an SOP

The template to design SOP is provided (Fig. 10.2).

1. **Introduction:**
   For the maintenance, safety, and integrity of the data archiving is an essential element of the Quality Management system. The systematic archiving of records smoothens the process and procedures of data retention and data retrieval.
2. **Purpose:**
   To manage the Archiving process in the laboratory
3. **Requirements:**

   (a) Termite free cabinets/Almirahs
   (b) Proper coding of the Cabinets, Documents, and researchers
   (c) Fireproof or Waterproof archiving cabinets or Almirahs
   (d) Proper Safety Management, e.g., Fire extinguisher or smoke alarm
   (e) Password-protected, or Lock-and-Key-protected documented places
   (f) Confidentiality of the records
   (g) Proper handover of duties to the other researcher or staff before leaving the laboratory
   (h) Approval from Study Director, Quality Assurance (QA) Personnel

4. **Procedure:**

   (a) Proper indexing and coding of the archiving document.
   (b) Well coded samples and proper compilation of the raw data and results of the study.
   (c) Proper validated data approved by the Study Director and QA.
   (d) Keeping of archiving data in termite free, rust free cabinet, Almirahs, and cupboards.
   (e) Archiving data kept in proper lockers with archivists.
   (f) Maintenance of data till the applicable retention period.
   (g) Retrieval of data from the archives and return back of data to archives should be properly reported.
   (h) Disposal of Archival data with the permission of Study Director and management.
   (i) Archivist must inform the Study Director when the archive procedure is done.

5. **Responsibility:**

   Personnel of the testing facility will be responsible to follow the SOP, and any deviation from the SOP should be intimated to Q.A. Person and/or Study Director.

   Status: The options include—Original Amended Revised Revalidated

   The particular option is chosen according to the current status of the SOP.

   Approvals: Approvals from the management, study director, and QA is required along with the signatures of the associated personnel.

	Name	Signature	Date
Author			
Q.A. Review			
Study Director			
Management Approval			

10.3 Purpose of Record Management

Documents are the key to govern any system or organization. Document control is the fundamental requirement in any office, institution, or lab for assuring data safety, security and confidentiality with an ethical code of conduct. Documents consist of informative data or evidence or records which may be on paper or recorded into an electronic device. These documents act as a manual to follow the guidelines of performing the experiment or to confirm the procedure to use [5].

In the current scenario, reliability, validity, reproducibility of the test data is required for worldwide acceptability as well as to get grants from the government

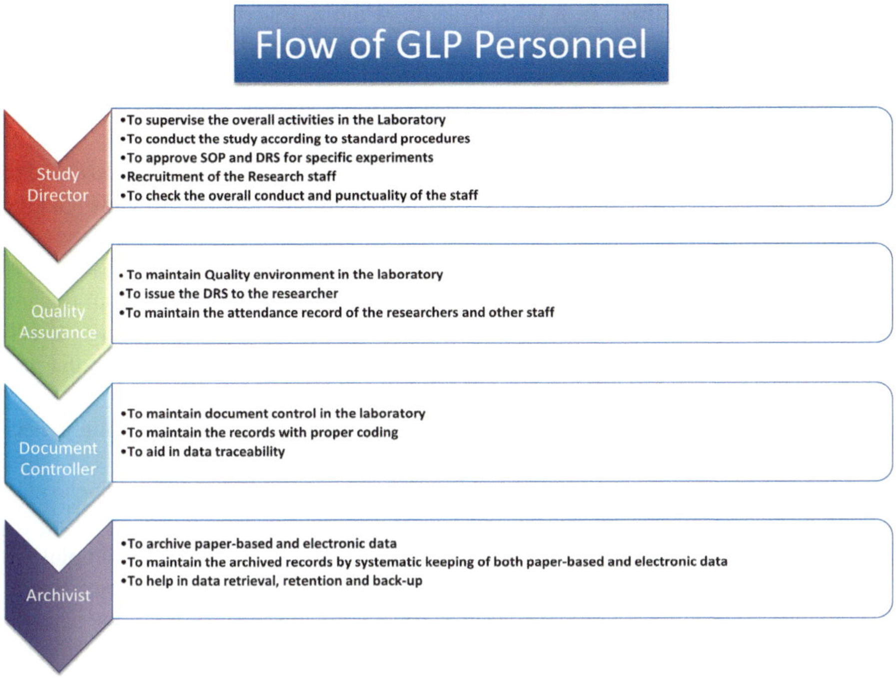

Fig. 10.3 Flow of GLP-oriented laboratories

and other funding agencies. GLP has the solution to all these current problems and is useful for future perspectives [6, 7]. The flow of the GLP personnel is shown in Fig. 10.3.

10.4 Best Practices for Record-Keeping and Preservation of Historical Records

The historical records can be preserved using the following best practices for document control:

1. **Coding of Documents:** Coding has an important role in the management of documents and archiving. By coding, we can find the documents easily, without wasting precious working hours. Many countries and Institutions emphasize on coding for better functioning. The current example is India, as the importance of coding is also highlighted in the New Education Policy (NEP) 2020. Coding is important not only to recognize the records in the lab but also for archiving the records. Coding makes the archiving process convenient for the students/ researchers. Coding should be done at various levels as follows:

(a) **Students Coding:** In a GLP system, when a student enters the lab, then Quality Assurance (QA) provides him/her with a unique student code so that they can maintain the records according to the number, and in the end, they can archive their documents according to the student code so that it can be found easily.
(b) **Room Coding:** If the lab is divided into chambers or rooms, it is essential to provide a room number. This ensures that the chambers/rooms can be located easily.
(c) **Cabinet Coding:** It is also necessary to provide a number to the cabinets in the room(R1, R2, R3, etc.). For proper management, first, add room no. and then cabinet no. For example, if room no. is 5 and cabinet belongs to R1, then the subcabinet no. will be 5R1. This will make it easier to find the particular place without describing it.
(d) **Equipment Coding :** To differentiate various equipment, its coding is necessary. Equipment coding may be according to Quality Assurance (QA) such as A1…A99 or AA…AZ then BA…BZ.
(e) **Sample Coding:** There should be well-designed coding so that the samples can be tracked easily. If a student with code 52 has collected the samples for his/her research work and the sample no. is YB-27, then the proper coding of the 52YB-27. This makes it easy to track the samples.
(f) **Documents Coding:** There are different types and formats of documents used in the lab or office. There are log sheets for different equipment, recurring and non-recurring material, and students' log register files. For example, on the cover page, the cabinet no. should be mentioned to locate it easily. In the equipment file, we can find the date of purchase or the calibration/service date. In the equipment log sheet, the researchers should enter the experiment date, name of the researcher, and the experiment performed.

2. **Data Recording Sheets**: Data recording sheets (DRS) are also very useful at the time of experiments. New researchers can easily perform the experiments in a stepwise manner, and if there is some new method required, then they can reschedule the step. It is very useful for future research.

10.5 Types of Documents and Their Management

1. The Standard Operating Procedure (SOPs), Data Repository System (DRS), Master Schedule, Indent register, Inventory and in account section the stock register, cash book, temperature log sheets, bill files (requisition file), reimbursement bills, correspondence files, salary registers are included in the documents in a research setting.
2. All the documents are approved by the Quality Assurance head (QA) and Personal Investigator (PI) of the Project.
3. All approved documents need to be well organized in a binded file and available for the staff or students to use, and blank forms must also be available there.

4. These forms and documents should also be available electronically, such as on a server or any lab network which acts as an interlink between the members of a lab or an Institute.
5. There should be an Index page that mentions about all the documents in the file, and it should be updated on a regular basis.
6. There should be a similar index on the cupboard or almirah, so that anyone is able to locate any concerned file easily.

All the documents should be attached in an appropriate manner in SOPs (Standard Operating Procedures). All documents should be approved by the head of the laboratories. The approved documents should be converted into electronic data and should be saved in the server. All forms should be bound in files. Division of the cabinet should be according to a unique number and the related file number. For example, the cabinet no. will be 5R1, if 5 is the room no., R is the whole cabinet, and 1 is the particular small subcabinet place.

10.6 Resources for Document Management

These include documents, email, digital imaging, softwares, record-keeping management services.

Data can be stored on paper or electronically.

1. **Paper Documents:** Paper documents include study plans, SOPs, DRSs, document files, ledger, letters, approvals, and notes on paper. It is an essential and commonly used process practiced everywhere by professionals. It should be well organized in a binded file. Electronic data hard copies are also considered as paper documents.
2. **Electronic Documents:** A popular phrase used in research is "increased complexity leads to decreased efficiency." GLP is an extraordinary way to manage and simplify all documents. Data stored on paper can be damaged or lost easily. To avoid these issues, it is important to save a copy of all the documents into the server and/or other devices. Electronic data can be stored in a CTMS software [8, 9]:

   CTMS Software: CTMS (Clinical Trial Management System) is a cost and time-effective software for clinical trials. It can track the pending tasks, database, and deadlines and store the information of participants. It can centralize the data without any delays [10].

10.7 Requirements for Electronic Data and Paper Data

Everything has its pros and cons. Electronic data is easily accessible, but sometimes it is very sensitive to access and store. Any defect in the system can destroy the whole data, hence the backups in drives are mandatory. However, both formats can be made compulsory. These methods of storing data are as shown (Table 10.1).

Table 10.1 Resources for document management

	Paper	Electronic
Requirements	• Plastic files or cobra files • All documents should be punched and kept in the files • Space and cupboards to keep the records	• CD • PD • Separate locked space in a computer
Approachability	GLP system should be followed to find any file easily	It should be well indexed
Security	• Cupboard should be free from termites and insects. • Need Lock and Key system for security of the documents	• It should be free from software viruses • Well spaced • Documents should be protected with passwords

10.8 The Role of Education and Training in Document Control and Archival of Records

In a GLP system, record management is a combination of various subjects. In a GLP-oriented lab, retention, privacy, and the archiving process should fulfil the mandates for GLP. All these should depend on the system and not on any person. In other words, document control should be system oriented and not person oriented. Even if the need to track a particular file arises after 20 years, one should be able to find it easily if the system is GLP oriented. For the proper record management and data archiving using GLP principles, education, and training are needed. In addition to this, the world is becoming digitalized. When everything came to a standstill due to the lockdown imposed due to the Covid-19 Pandemic, Technology came in as a savior. Education, business, official work, etc., continued virtually, and this promoted sustainable development. In the modern era, new technology is being used to manage records, hence being up to date becomes all the more important, for which regular training programs should be held.

10.9 Common Problems in Document Control and Archiving Records

As we know, document control is a complicated process without GLP management. Challenges can arise while managing both electronic as well as hard copy data (Table 10.2).

Table 10.2 Common problems related to electronic and hard copy data

Common problems in document control	Electronic data	Hard copy paper data
Insufficient storage	It is a common challenge in the management of electronic data. To avoid these issues, clean the junk file on time and archive the files which are not in use	It is also a great challenge in the lab due to limited space
Susceptibility to damage	CD, Pen drives are easily accessible, but these items are susceptible to damage by water, fire, and dust granules	Paper data is susceptible to damage by water, fire, moisture, and insects
Limitations	There is a limit to the amount of data that can be stored in each drive. However, we can improve this after spending some funds	Insufficient Storage capacity is also a challenge here. Although it can be improved, it is very costly compared to electronic data management. A new room or cabinet also needs to be hired for the same

10.10 Data Recording Sheet (DRS)

The data recording sheets, popularly known as DRS, are the main requisite of GLP systems. DRS plays an imperative role in maintaining the authenticity of the experiment. It also mentions the correct way to conduct a particular experiment sequentially. DRS should mirror what has been done in that particular experiment. The result, any mishappening or mistake related to the failed experiments can also be reported. Some features of DRS are illustrated (Fig. 10.4) and explained below :

1. **Indexing:** The DRS should have a proper index, and a separate file of each student with a proper student code. The indexing facilitates the traceability of the particular DRS using date and sample number.
2. **Location:** The DRS needs to be properly kept with the QA personnel. The maintenance of DRS should be done by the QA personnel with proper indexing on the particular cabinet, almirah, or safe so that it is easily traceable. Moreover, it should not disturb the arrangement of the previous records kept there. There needs to be interconnectivity within the different records, so that when there is any kind of ambiguity, it can be sorted. The QA is required to keep the records safe using proper lock and key or password.
3. **Issuance of DRS:** The DRS are issued by the QA. There needs to be a proper time period for DRS issuance. Moreover, issuance of the DRS is subject to the return of the previously issued DRS duly signed by the study director.

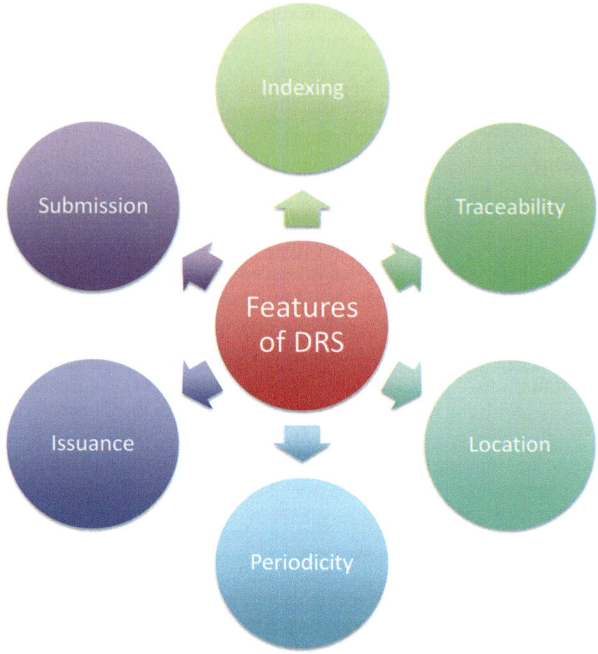

Fig. 10.4 Features of Data Recording Sheets (DRS)

10.11 GLP for Maintaining Records and Document Control

The responsibility to manage GLP using proper records lies with the Quality Assurance personnel. The Quality Assurance (QA) personnel plays a prominent role in the GLP system.

1. **Control of Attendance:** The QA has the responsibility to maintain the attendance of the research staff, hence maintaining punctuality in the research lab. Punctuality helps in time management and timely completion of various research projects.
2. **Control of Movement:** In a GLP-compliant lab, it is important to control the movement of the research staff. It is essential to maintain the productivity of the work, especially in times like the COVID-19 pandemic.
3. **Meeting Minutes:** A number of meetings are held in the laboratory to get updates on various assignments from the research staff. Therefore, noting down lab meeting minutes is an important process for document control. It eventually aids in the researchers' growth.
4. **Prevention of Inventory Pilferage:** For protection from any type of pilferage in the laboratory, the inventories need to be safeguarded with password-protected lockers or proper lock and key. The key of the inventories must be with an authorized person. A proper issuance register of the keys should be maintained, which contains the signature of the concerned person to whom the keys were issued. Moreover, the responsibility of maintenance of the inventories in the laboratory

can be distributed among the researchers. Additionally, password-protected doors in the lab are also helpful in inhibiting entry to outsiders in the laboratory environment.

5. **Monitor the Use of Resources :** The resources and the infrastructure are a very important aspect of GLP. To check or monitor the usage of resources, different kit log sheets are maintained. The log sheets with Log sheet no. are used, and the users make an entry on a particular log sheet of the specific chemical with date, amount used, and balance quality.

10.12 Electronic Records and Its Management

The twenty-first century is the era of modern technology. Technology has played a major role in many fields, including research. There are various instruments, which are based on computer systems for conducting experiments and recording data, for e.g., RT-PCR, gradient-PCR, UV-Spectrophotometer, Nano-Doppler, Ph meters, and ELISA readers. The maintenance and management of electronic data is an important aspect of document control. Electronic data is the need of the hour. It is very important to control the electronic data records by preparing better backups, having a proper antivirus, and a computer protection with passwords. In the GLP system, electronic data is very important to generate and preserve so that it can be retrieved anytime. The physical records have some disadvantages like susceptibility to damage by physical factors, but electronic records may even be re-used. Electronic records are prepared directly on the computer system using different softwares like Microsoft word, Microsoft excel, Powerpoint, Adobe pdf, Google docs, etc. The data related to the study can be electronically recorded by the primary observations in the computerized systems [11].

Moreover, the storage of data in electronic records is eco-friendly. It is a requisite of the GLP system to maintain a proper electronic record of the pen–paper-based data or the data available in hard copies. It is important to note that the raw data collected on paper needs to be properly converted into electronic form through proper computerized systems. The collection of raw data should be carried out properly following the GLP guidelines under the strict instructions of the study director. According to OECD (2018), for the maintenance of data in the form of electronic records, properly equipped computerized systems are required with proper planning, performing monitoring, recording, and archiving as shown in Fig. 10.5 [12].

10.12.1 Prerequisites for Electronic Data

There are some prerequisites for preparing and maintaining electronic records, especially when using computerized systems. These are permanence, security, backups, password protection with limited access to the people, and traceability. There should be a proper backup system available in case the present system stops working due to any problem. Moreover, system security is also an important issue,

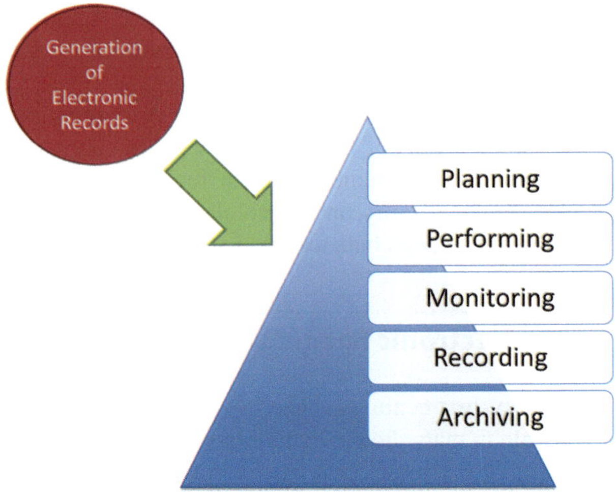

Fig. 10.5 The methods for generating electronic records [12]

which needs to be dealt with, as only limited people should have access to the data. A password-protected system helps in better document control. Data traceability is also a major aspect of electronic control. We should be able to trace the data whenever we need it, in a systematic and smooth manner [1]. For electronic management of the records, it is necessary that the database is organized in a logical and systematic manner for it to be accessible and traceable. This can be done by making a proper archiving folder in the computer systems with password protection. It further helps in tracing months or years old data with proper details like date, specimen, and personnel. In GLP-oriented lab facilities, if host services are being used for the maintenance of electronic records, then an agreement mentioning proper terms and conditions needs to be signed by both sides [13].

10.12.2 Precautions for Storing Electronic Data

The storage of data in electronic records has its advantages as well as disadvantages. However, by adopting some preventive measures, its disadvantages can be overcome. The person who is handling or maintaining the electronic data must have expertise in using computerized systems. Moreover, the person also needs to have expertise in dealing with unfavorable situations in handling the data, for e.g., knowledge of backups. The computerized systems need to be accessible only to a limited number of designated people [14]. The computerized systems need to be well equipped, validated, secure, maintained, and operated in the GLP-oriented labs. In the GLP-oriented labs, the whole management system assures the authenticity and data recording in computerized systems [14]. The whole computerized system is well connected with the server with a high-speed Internet connectivity. Calibration of hardware and upgradation of the software should be done regularly and on time.

There should be proper indexing and coding of different folders along with a separate archiving folder in the system.

10.13 Archival of Records

Archival is an important component of data management and helps in maintaining the data integrity and safety of the records. Archiving involves storing the data from the main working place to other safe areas in order to retain them. Data is stored in a secure area that is fully dedicated for archiving purposes where all types of documents can be stored which are not being currently used. The same process as previously discussed for proper management of paper data and electronic records is also applicable in archiving. Although there are certain differences between paper data and electronic data archiving, yet there are some fundamental similarities. To manage all types of records and materials, there should be an archivist, who is responsible for archiving all the data as suggested by the study investigator or/and Quality assurance head in that appropriate place (Archiving place) [11].

To make the process of retrieval easier, there should be proper Indexing. It should also be ensured that the movement of records and archives is properly controlled [15].

10.13.1 Access to the Archive

To increase efficiency, accountability, and transparency, access to the archiving process should be properly documented, and every visit should be recorded in a GLP system. The indexing should remain unchanged at that time [16].

10.13.2 Records to Be Retained

The following documents need to be retained:

Study proposal, approval of IEC, raw data (including all DRS's SOP'S and student raw registers, log registers, validation sheets), Old bill files, attendance registers, students registers, including all data into pen drives, all QA sheets, master schedules of previous years, etc.

10.13.3 Procedure to Archive

The responsibilities of an archivist have been discussed, but the study director is mainly responsible for data integrity. The archivist can archive the records after approval. The study director is responsible for ensuring that records are archived on time and for deciding where, when, what, how to archive [17].

10.13.4 Format of Archiving

To make it traceable and to make the retention process easy, we should follow some important steps, and coding is one of them. Coding plays an important role in archiving the paper data. The coding of archiving rooms, cabinets, students, and documents is essential to make the process of tracing the documents easy. Coding has an important role in the management of documents and archiving, as it helps to find the right location without wasting precious working hours.

10.13.5 Benefits of Proper Archiving

(a) It makes the compliance process easy.
(b) It manages the space for proper files.
(c) Recovery makes easier after the document control.
(d) It assures the backup of all documents.
(e) It secures disaster recovery.
(f) It makes a strong connection between the Documents, so it is also helpful in Collaborations [17].

10.14 Electronic Data Archiving

To manage all the documents which are not being used very frequently, it is better to convert them into electronic documents via scanning and then archive them into secure systems. This is called Electronic Data Management System (EDMS). In fact, all the essential lab paper documents can be converted into electronic documents and be saved into a server or any other device, so that the authorized personnel can retrieve them easily [18] . This also helps to lessen the burden of excessive paperwork. Many labs are now archiving data using electronic means. Although electronic archiving has a tremendous role in the management of data, it may also create some difficulties in tracking if not properly arranged. The records have to be divided into categories according to the information or depending on the nature of the activity. Staff and students may find it difficult to switch to electronic archiving, so appropriate training must be provided for this [8].

10.14.1 Standard Operating Procedures of Archiving Electronic Records

Electronic records are easy to create but a little hard to maintain. To make the electronic data achieving process easier, some standards should be followed.

Electronic records should be safely stored in pen drives, CDs, or optical disks in order to physically archive these items. These records should be placed at an appropriate place for electronic devices, i.e., the area should be free from magnetic fields and moisture.

It is necessary to have a backup of the same records in two different devices, i.e., in CDs and pen drives both [18–20]. If we are archiving data into the system, then it has to be stored in a secure place protected with passwords, so that no one can change or delete it.

The IT sector is rapidly advancing, so there is a need for time to time upgradation of the archive facilities according to modern advancements.

Remember that all the "electronic data archiving" operations should be performed under the guidance of an archivist. It is important that an Archivist is well versed with information technology, so that he can handle every electronic operation [11]. Electronic records are very sensitive, hence there is a basic need to examine the records from time to time. If there is any missing record in any of the devices, it has to be copied from another device without any delay. If both electronic devices have lost the data, then data should be taken from the hard copies, and backup should be created again in the electronic devices with the help of imaging techniques or scanning techniques. All these operations should be properly documented under the QA and/or the Study director [11, 12, 17, 18].

10.14.2 Benefits of Electronic Archiving

Electronic archiving ensures that :

1. The data is protected and can be maintained easily.
2. Data is easily traceable.
3. The extra burden of paperwork is reduced.
4. Storage and management of data are cost effective.

10.15 Future Directions and Clinical Implications

A lack of proper documentation practices is one of the most common findings during on-site inspections [21]. The documentation should be such that an independent observer should be able to reconstruct the whole process using the documents [21]. As mentioned by FDA, Good documentation should follow the principle of ALCOA-attributable, legible, contemporaneous, original, and accurate [22]. According to ICH–GCP guidelines for clinical trials, data is saved in a Trial Master File, which is then archived [23]. With the advent of digitization, software-based methods of document control and archiving have been developed. CTMS (Clinical Trial Management system) software are being used by pharmaceutical companies and CROs, but its extension to academic Institutions also can make communication and tracking of data easier, and improve efficiency, especially for multicenter trials, provided the privacy and security of data are taken care of [24]. For the appropriate management of data in the contemporary era, it is important for the person managing it to be up to date with newer technology. Developing an SOP for documentation, adequate training regarding GLP and GCP, and understanding the process of documentation can improve the documentation quality and the process as a whole [21].

10.16 Conclusion

In the GLP environment, document control and archiving records are the backbone of administration and other research-related work. It secures the data of different types of studies/researches and assures the retention and retrieval period having proper documentation practices. It prepares one to face any type of challenges their academic career such as allegations on research, thesis defense, warning notices by the funding/approval agencies in the future, even after many years. This chapter summarizes the role of document control and the importance of archiving records in management, and the use of standard operating procedures. This chapter aims to provide the solutions to common problems in paper data and electronic data archiving and management. It has evaluated all the aspects regarding data and how to archive it. DRSs, SOPs, the formats and methods of archiving, and best record-keeping practices in GLP management have also been described. This chapter will encourage the labs/offices to move towards electronic data management and Good documentation practices in the GLP system. Future directions in this digital era lie in the advancement of the labs to adopt the above suggestions, methods, and systems in their administrative work to improve the quality of data.

References

1. World Health Organization. Laboratory Quality Management System Training Toolkit. [Internet] 2020. https://www.who.int/ihr/training/laboratory_quality/16_b_content_doc_rec.pdf?ua=1. Accessed 26 Nov 2020.
2. OECD. Series on principles of good laboratory practice and compliance monitoring no 15: establishment and control of archives that operate in compliance with the principles of GLP; 2007. http://www.oecd.org/officialdocuments/publicdisplaydocumentpdf/?doclanguage=en&cote=env/jm/mono(2007)10. Accessed 26 Nov 2020.
3. FDA. CFR—Code of Federal Regulations Title 21. Updated Apr 2020. https://www.accessdata.fda.gov/scripts/cdrh/cfdocs/cfcfr/CFRSearch.cfm?CFRPart=820
4. World Health Organization. 2013. https://www.who.int/immunization/programmes_systems/supply_chain/EVM_model_SOP_manual_EN_June_2013_compact.pdf. Accessed 27 Nov 2020.
5. Asmoro D. Control of Documents and records [Internet]. https://www.academia.edu/30252173/CONTROL_OF_DOCUMENTS_AND_RECORDS. Accessed 27 Nov 2020.
6. Jena GB, Chavan S. Implementation of good laboratory practices (GLP) in basic scientific research: translating the concept beyond regulatory compliance. Regul Toxicol Pharmacol. 2017;89:20–5.
7. Grainger LA, Ferries R. Lab design best practices-design document. Albuquerque, NM: Sandia National Lab; 2013.
8. Gupta SK. Paperless clinical trials: myth or reality? Indian J Pharmacol. 2015;47(4):349.

9. Rotenstreich S. The difference between electronic and paper documents. The George Washington University. https://www2.seas.gwu.edu/~shmuel/WORK/Differences/Chapter%203%20-%20Sources.pdf. Accessed 27 Nov 2020
10. Choi B, Drozdetski S, Hackett M, Lu C, Rottenberg C, Yu L, et al. Usability comparison of three clinical trial management systems. AMIA Annu Symp Proc. 2005;2005:921.
11. World Health Organization. GLP Trainer. https://www.who.int/tdr/publications/documents/glp-trainer.pdf. Accessed 29 Nov 2020.
12. OECD. Storage and retention of records and materials. In: Guidance document on good in vitro method practices (GIVIMP). Paris: OECD; 2018. https://doi.org/10.1787/9789264304796-15-en.
13. OECD. Good laboratory practice: frequently asked questions (FAQ) [Internet]. http://www.oecd.org/chemicalsafety/testing/glp-frequently-asked-questions.htm. Accessed 28 Nov 2020.
14. Food and Drug Administration. Guidance for industry: part 11, electronic records; electronic signatures—scope and application. Washington, DC: US Department of Health and Human Services; 2003.
15. Sun HL, Wei ZH. Documentation archiving in clinical data management. Yao xuexuebao = Acta Pharmaceutica Sinica. 2015;50(11):1410–4.
16. Vines TH, Andrew RL, Bock DG, Franklin MT, Gilbert KJ, Kane NC, et al. Mandated data archiving greatly improves access to research data. FASEB J. 2013;27(4):1304–8.
17. Whitlock MC. Data archiving in ecology and evolution: best practices. Trends Ecol Evol. 2011;26(2):61–5.19.
18. Working Group on Information Technology (AGIT). Good laboratory practice (GLP); Guidelines for the archiving of electronic raw data in a GLP Environment. Qual Assur J. 2003;7(4):262–9.
19. Kuchinke W, Aerts J, Semler SC, Ohmann C. CDISC standard-based electronic archiving of clinical trials. Methods Inf Med. 2009;48(05):408–13.
20. Kauffmann HM, Kamp H, Fuchs R, Chorley BN, Deferme L, Ebbels T, Hackermüller J, Perdichizzi S, Poole A, Sauer UG, Tollefsen KE. Framework for the quality assurance of 'omics technologies considering GLP requirements. Regul Toxicol Pharmacol. 2017;91:S27–35.
21. Bargaje C. Good documentation practice in clinical research. Perspect Clin Res. 2011;2(2):59–63.
22. Food and Drug Administration. Guidance for industry: computerized systems used in clinical investigations; 2007.
23. ICH. International conference on harmonisation of technical requirements for registration of pharmaceuticals for human use; 2015. www.ich.org
24. Park YR, Yoon YJ, Koo HY, Yoo S, Choi CM, Beck SH, et al. Utilization of a clinical trial management system for the whole clinical trial process as an integrated database: system development. J Med Internet Res. 2018;20(4):e103.

Academic Social Responsibility and Quality Assurance in the Developing World: A Framework for Implementation

11

Avijit Banik and Avik Mitra

11.1 Introduction

Corporate Social Responsibility (CSR), over the years, has become a successful concept for companies and industries in order to ensure their capacity for long-term value creation and gain in competitive markets, while this sense of responsibility remains mostly isolated in policies and guidelines in academic settings without much into practice. In developing countries, researchers and academicians are mostly found working in isolation, limiting their important findings and practices without embedding them into a larger goal for social benefits. While many times their groundbreaking works are made available as a piece of publication in the scientific domain, they fail to connect to the common people's need and welfare. Though scientists are bound by the act of "responsible conduct of research" but they need to rise above their limited ethical responsibilities and pursue a broader and larger social requirement of their body of work, termed as Scientific Social Responsibility or Academic Social Responsibility (ASR) [1].

Corporate Social Responsibility (CSR) is a dominant theme for decades in the world of business. Despite the practical dissimilarities, parallel to the corporate world, the scientific world also poses similar challenges such as ethical governance of Institutions, respecting culture and values, balancing between self and societal interests and justifying self and outside regulation [1]. The term Academic Social Responsibility (ASR) can be defined as the means of integrating social values in the higher academic Institutes to not confine them to learning alone but to disseminate

A. Banik (✉)
Department of Pharmacology and Chemical Biology, Emory University School of Medicine, Atlanta, GA, USA
e-mail: avibanik@yahoo.co.in

A. Mitra
National Board for Quality Promotion, Quality Council of India, New Delhi, India

A. Anand (ed.), *Quality Assurance Implementation in Research Labs*,
https://doi.org/10.1007/978-981-16-3074-3_11

the power of learning for societal benefits. Recently, the concept is getting embedded in many academic Institutes, including research establishments, as a potential way to sustain the progress towards value addition in the respective fields. The purpose of ASR is to achieve sustainability blended with ethical responsibilities towards the immediate society for improved health and livelihood [2]. It is believed that the larger vision and mission of a teaching and research Institute should focus on how it can contribute to the welfare of society form where it draws funds to sustain their activities. Though widely deliberated and partly practiced in developed countries, the concept is yet to be defined within the ambit of academic Institutes, making it necessary to develop steps for implementing ASR in the context of an academic Institute in the developing world.

11.2 Role of United States in Steering Academic Social Responsibility (ASR)

After World War II, the United Nations in the 1948 General Assembly paved the way for the Universal Declaration of Human Rights, depicting liberty, security, and well-being of human lives through social justice of equality [3]. The Association of Academic Health Centers (AAHC), founded in 1969, is one of the pioneering elements in America's health care system by educating and training next-generation medical practitioners towards advancing global health and well-being of the communities [4]. AAHC represents a large body of member Institutions, including allied health, public health, dentistry, nursing, pharmacy, veterinary and graduate schools. Through their well-constructed campaigns, AAHC has spearheaded the nationwide movement to inculcate the importance of social determinants in the healthcare system. While the value of ASR is very much at the core of medical fraternities in the USA, it lacked altruistic enactment due to Institutional structure, regulation, and accreditation. An incentivized system and the "guild mentality" of the health care professionals have limited AAHC's efforts of infusing ASR into a nationwide movement [5].

The "guild mentality" largely divides the health care practitioners between medicine and public health. It leads to competition and duplication without considering the patient community as a partner. Another barrier is the larger divide within the health care professionals among the disciplines inside the academic Institutes. This inhibits the interaction between different disciplines, obstructing the collaboration across schools and departments. Competition within faculties and reserving skill-sets within the departments also add to this nature of silo. Evaluation and promotion of the faculties are mostly based on publication and revenue records without giving much importance to the collaborative efforts and societal contribution [6]. Unfortunately, being a first-world country, the US health care system is still driven by profit margins with health insurance programs and does not advocate for equality for social well-being among different strata of economic divisions in the society [7].

Despite such challenges and limitations in the system, the value of social responsibility is embodied in different public and private institutes of excellence. One such study reveals how social accountability is conceptualized as a core value in a Nursing School of a private Institute and implemented into their curriculum. Funded fellowship programs focusing on leadership and social responsibility are awarded to deserving students. As a part of their curriculum, students are allowed to work closely with the underprivileged population in clinical settings. Through journaling, debriefing, and other collaborations, students analyze the broader social issues related to inequality, human rights, and poverty [8]. In fact, a recent study scored more than sixty thousand physicians linked to the American Medical Association (AMA) based on their placement in primary care settings, distribution to underserved areas, and if they belong to the underrepresented minorities in the US medical schools. Interestingly, three historically black colleges and universities ranked high on this social mission score. Public and community-based medical schools scored higher than noncommunity private schools [9].

11.3 Global Status of ASR in the Developing World

The ISO Strategic Advisory Group, an international body, recommending and advocating for social, ethical standards in world business, notes that Social Responsibility is "a balanced approach for organizations to address economic, social and environmental issues in a way that aims to benefit people, communities and society" [10]. Although this definition is a benchmark targeted at the corporate world, one cannot deny the relative significance of these values in the academic and scientific paradigm. In 1998, The UNESCO organized the World Conference on Higher Education in Paris where the committee announced "The World Declaration on Higher Education in the Twenty-First Century" and in the following year introduced the ambitious policy document called "Bologna Declaration" to make higher education accessible and comparable within countries across Europe. The Ministry of education from 29 European countries adopted this declaration. Subsequently, this declaration was amended several times based on the evolving needs, and in the 2009 accord, it acknowledged the need for social responsibility in the Universities, highlighting it as an intrinsic factor of the higher education system [11]. Despite several challenges of expansion, globalization, corporatization, and political skewness faced by Institutes of higher education, the European Universities of eminence are largely imbibed by the Magna Charta Universitatum, the declaration of the Bologna Process to accommodate the concept of social responsibilities into higher education [11].

Medical education is an area where ASR plays an indispensable role in dwelling with ethics to sustain and improve equity in the health care system. Latin American countries such as Mexico, Chile, and Brazil have substantially expanded economically in the recent decades, and that has led to a surge in the induction of many medical and health care Institutes in these countries. A qualitative analysis between Latin American and non-Latin American countries reveals the existence of ASR by principle in most of the medical schools reviewed in the study, but the implementation was poor in Latin American schools as the concept of ASR was not well practiced during training [12]. There is much debate over the extent of adoption of the concept of social responsibilities as a part of the curriculum, but it is widely acknowledged that a proper framework of implementation is necessary to overcome the health disparities in medical schools [13, 14]. The WHO recommendations, way back in 1995, highlight the need for social accountability in medical schools in order to shape the future health system and to justify financial funding through public taxes. WHO recognizes the four major pillars such as relevance, quality, cost-effectiveness, and equity in health care, for implementing social accountability in the Institutions [14]. The sub-Saharan countries, in particular, South Africa, has a long history of practicing "humanness," in a local language called, "Ubuntu" encouraging societal well-being among its citizens. Likewise, medical schools in this region are also influenced by the "Ubuntu" effect, and over the decades, through several recommendations such as The 1988 Edinburgh Declaration, the 1995 Cape Town Declaration, implemented the elements of social responsibilities in their policies and practices [15].

11.4 ASR in India: More in Policies than in Practice?

India's scientific community has mostly followed a prototype of western countries such as the Code of Nuremberg (1947) and later the Declaration of Helsinki (1964) as a point of reference for the responsible conduct of biomedical research. However, these policies have driven the scientists and researchers more towards patients' safety than connecting to their larger societal benefits. The Indian Council of Medical Research (ICMR) has had its own Ethical Guidelines for Biomedical and Health Research for long but it only recently includes the importance of social value incorporating the sense of social responsibilities in health research among the stakeholders [16]. There is at least a paradigm shift in the current scientific atmosphere in India where the scientific community and the governmental bodies are deliberating on the value of social benefits for a larger community and should not be looked as "leftover-benefits" from the study outcomes [17]. There are isolated reports also suggesting the need of implementing ASR in the framework of medical colleges in India by raising above the ethics of patient care [18].

In 2019, the Ministry of Science and Technology under the Indian Government had released a draft policy (see http://go.nature.com/32sihv2) for public consultation on Scientific Social Responsibility (SSR). It aims further consultation, discussion, and debates to shorten the gaps between science and society in our ecosystem. The Science and Engineering Research Board (SERB), under Govt. of India, is on the verge of implementing this policy soon. When effective, it will require the researchers to spend a minimum of 10 days/year in public engagement through sharing their knowledge and resources to the community, and the credit for SSR efforts will be a part of their evaluation process. It is proposed that each institute will have their autonomous SSR implementation and monitoring system and would publish an annual report on SSR activities within the institute. The policy acknowledges several social benefits out of this engagement, such as encouraging the next generation for science and technology education, upbringing neighboring scientific community by knowledge and resource sharing, improving the productivity of MMSE/Startups by technical support, and empowering weaker and neglected sections of our society through scientific solutions [19, 20].

Because of the structure of the current curriculum and the condescending attitude of academicians, they are largely found skipping their societal responsibilities and community development initiatives. A recent case study on the engagement of academic scientists from a medical institute in Northern India highlights the benefit of their social outreach initiatives. A group of researchers has dedicated 2 hours every week for close to 5 years to a campus health hygiene initiative under the purview of the Clean India Movement (Swachh Bharat Abhiyan), a Govt. initiative to engage its citizens in the community sanitation drive. The efforts from this group of academicians have led to improving awareness on hygienic practices among the common public, reduced littering, and a cleaner campus. This initiative has even drawn prestigious awards to the Institute, as the cleanest hospital in the country [21]. This study sets an example of how a case of ASR in academic setting plays a significant role in not only transforming the community, but also in inspiring the academicians towards nation-building [22]. This report highlights that the outcomes are prominent, and only Institutional remodeling is required to inculcate such practices into the curriculum effectively. It is imperative to mention that when the current SSR policy by SERB will be incorporated into the Indian academic settings, a tangible framework for implementation should be in place to materialize the beneficial outcomes of such policies.

11.5 Framework for Implementation of ASR in Indian Academics

While the term Corporate Social Responsibility (CSR) is not new for business organizations across the world, the term Academic Social Responsibility (ASR) is fairly new for academic Institutes both in developing countries as well as in India. Business looks at CSR from the viewpoint for value creation for its stakeholders and also considers it as an important pillar for building competitive advantage.

Academics, on the other hand, are yet to get a clear understanding of the implications of ASR for stakeholders like faculty, students, employees, fund providers, government, community, etc. Since businesses started committing itself to CSR, various methodologies and approaches for implementing CSR have developed over the years. Looking at the wide interest in CSR, the International Organization for Standardization (ISO) also came out with ISO26000 guidance standard on social responsibility. The standards helped the business to use it as a tool to integrate, implement and promote social responsibility through its policies and practices. Though there was no such guidance available for ASR, some of the implementation practices of CSR were found to be equally useful for ASR. These were as under:

1. Commitment and direction setting
2. Self-assessment or self-diagnosis

3. Presentation of findings
4. Reporting and communication

Commitment is essential to direct the efforts of the academic community towards social responsibility. Commitment is demonstrated through the formation of a team comprising of members both from within the campus as well as external members. This team will need to work with a diverse group of stakeholders and work on the following:

1. To develop a self-assessment or a self-diagnostic tool.
2. To identify areas where ASR practices can be initiated.
3. To suggest areas of improvement.
4. To link academic processes with socially responsible projects.
5. To develop an appropriate reporting and communication plan of ASR practices to different stakeholders through different channels like social media, website, etc.

In the self-assessment or self-diagnostic phase, the aim will be to determine where the academic Institute stands with respect to ASR. All the team members will be involved in this exercise, and it can be conducted through various research methods like surveys, interviews, focus group discussions, etc. This self-assessment will highlight issues like how the Institute should be organized to become a socially responsible Institution, how it should interact with society for promoting sustainable human development, etc.

The presentation of the findings will include the presentation of data, survey results, interview reviews, opinions, and suggestions that will be obtained during the self-diagnosis phase. The findings should also include the main results, the selection of projects for ASR and the improvement needed in different areas.

Reporting is the key element of this process. The report will include results of self-diagnosis, actions developed, projects identified and implemented, recommendations for future work, etc. The report has to be communicated to different stakeholders.

11.6 Steps in ASR Implementation

Every organization has to actually develop its own steps for implementation, which will depend on its context as determined by several internal and external issues like legal, financial, social, etc. However, since ASR can be considered as a new or change initiative, the well-formulated steps tested in CSR like, Plan-Do-Study-Act (P-D-S-A) may be used as a framework on which activities are needed for ASR can be established. The P-D-S-A cycle was developed by Deming to turn ideas into actions and actions into learnings [23–25]. The cycle of P-D-S-A can be classically defined as:

Table 11.1 Organizational phases of ASR implementation based on P-D-S-A cycle

Phases	Main activities	Associated tasks (indicative only)
Plan	• Decide on the aims and objectives of the intervention • Decide on the best method to achieve the above • Decide on the strategy to be deployed	• Form ASR team • Build support of all identified stakeholders and employees • Conduct an ASR assessment to define the change/intervention required • Study what others are doing • Decide on direction, scope, roles, and responsibilities for ASR implementation
Do	• Implement ASR • Plan of implementation	• Conduct training for assessment • Develop a necessary communication plan • Document the problems encountered and other unexpected outcomes • Start the process of analysis of data • Measure achievement against what had been planned
Study	• Summarize what has been learnt	• Complete the data analysis • Measure the progress achieved • Summarize learnings including recommendations • Report the findings to all stakeholders
Act	• Act on the changes/ improvements needed in the Plan	• Start implementing the next cycle of ASR plan

- **Plan**: Define the change or intervention required.
- **Do**: Carry out the change or intervention.
- **Study**: Collect and analyze the information on the change, intervention carried out, and the outcome.
- **Act:** Use this knowledge to recommend and revise the plan as necessary.

Based on the P-D-S-A phases, the implementation framework is structured in detail in Table 11.1.

This framework is intended to help the management of any academic Institute to assess its effect on society and accordingly make it a part of the decision-making process. It is to be understood that the ASR approach should be an integrated part of the strategic management process.

11.7 ASR as Part of a Strategic Planning Process

The strategic planning process (including academic Institutes) helps the organization to develop its vision for the future. Hence, it is imperative that ASR is made part of the strategic planning process. This will facilitate in the following aspects:

(a) Focusing on agreed upon activities of ASR
(b) Improving the effectiveness of ASR outcomes
(c) Identifying the internal changes that are required in the organization/institute

(d) Improving the commitment towards ASR
(e) Increasing value creation of the institute, especially among the community and society
(f) Helping in the development of sustained competitive advantage

It is, however, important to remember that each Institute has to work out its own strategic plan and the manner in which it wants to integrate ASR within its plan.

11.8 Integrating ASR in the Strategic Planning Process

11.8.1 Understand How the Organization Views ASR

There is a need to integrate ASR into the vision and mission of the organization. This is because it significantly contributes towards building a positive image and enhance the trust of the community. It also establishes credibility among the stakeholders. This understanding is essential for an Institute to behave in a socially responsible manner.

11.8.2 Understand Stakeholders' Strategic Needs and Desires

Any credible ASR will encourage involvement from the stakeholders. In order to make the ASR initiative realistic and achievable, stakeholders' needs and desires are to be thoroughly understood. Ineffective stakeholders' engagement may lead to conflicts later on. Not identifying what is important to your stakeholders will adversely impact the success of the initiative.

11.8.3 Determine How ASR Is Vital to the Organization's Vision and Mission

Being a voluntary initiative, ASR may not get due importance until and unless it is included in the vision and mission of the Institute. The leadership team of an Institute must devote time and effort to determining the role of ASR in the vision and mission statements. The outcome of such an effort will be a steady commitment towards social responsibility and would facilitate changes required for implementing ASR.

11.8.4 Recognize and Utilize Quality Management Methods

To put an ASR in place, an Institute would need the following to be put in place:

(a) A sustainable management system
(b) A performance framework
(c) A continuous improvement program

The quality management principles, methods, practices, and tools will go a long way to achieve the above.

11.8.5 Commit to Internal Assessment Methods to Know the Effectiveness of Actions

The first step towards monitoring the progress of ASR is to develop and commit towards an internal assessment method within the organization which would be carried out periodically. The assessment results will provide critical inputs to understand the effectiveness of the ASR initiative.

11.8.6 Embrace a Framework or Management System Regarding Tactical Planning for ASR

A tactical plan will outline what each department/functional area of an Institute needs to achieve, how it must do so, and who has the responsibility for implementation, all with reference to ASR. Management system refers to a set of policies, processes, and procedures to facilitate the achievement of a project's objectives. A management system framework helps in a tactical planning process.

11.9 Need for Quality Assurance in Implementing ASR

Since P-D-S-A can be utilized for the implementation of ASR, it is important to develop a quality assurance plan for effective implementation. The quality assurance plan, in fact, establishes the criteria, tools, and procedures for monitoring the processes of implementation in line with the aims and objectives, methodologies, timelines, budget, etc. A good quality assurance plan will define roles and responsibilities, the methods to assure quality, actions necessary for the management of deviation from the goals, and to track and report progress [26]. Once the Institute decides to implement ASR, it becomes important that it addresses the quality assurance requirements at the design and development phase as well as the implementation stage of ASR. This approach will ensure community engagement and collaboration at every stage of ASR implementation.

11.10 Future Directions and Clinical Implications

It is understood that the Academic Social Responsibilities (ASR) or Scientific Social Responsibilities (SSR) are included in the policies in many countries around the globe, but a proper framework of implementation is widely lacking. Sometimes, these social values are overlooked at individual levels at the Institutes due to political interference, profit-driven curriculum, vagueness in social vision, and condescending attitudes of academicians. Therefore, all of the above contributing factors must be addressed in order to implement the value of ASR in achieving a positive impact on the academic settings. While more studies are warranted to examine the relationship of the social determinants with community benefits, it is clear that increased openness, training, knowledge, and resource sharing in the workforce will induce the elements of social values in the mind of academicians. The clinical implications of ASR in the medical Institutes are largely associated with the health care system and its valued services. It is beyond doubt that a proper implementation of ASR into medical academics will induce long-term social benefits through a renewed work ethics. It should be more in practice than in policies, if the country thrives to develop a value-driven system rather than profit-driven corporations in healthcare for the upcoming generation.

References

1. Conley JM, Munoz G, Prince AER, Davis AM, Cadigan RJ. Scientific social responsibility: lessons from the corporate social responsibility movement. Am J Bioeth. 2015;15(12):64–6.
2. Krogsgaard-Larsen P, Thostrup P, Besenbacher F. Scientific social responsibility: a call to arms. Angew Chem Int Ed Engl. 2011;50(46):10738–40.
3. General Assembly of the United Nations. Universal Declaration of Human Rights [Internet]; 1948. http://www.un.org/Overview/rights.html. Accessed 29 Nov 2020.
4. Karpf M. The role of academic health centers in addressing health equity and social determinants of health. Acad Med. 2019;94(9):1273–5.
5. Wartman SA, Steinberg MJ. The role of academic health centers in addressing social responsibility. Med Teach. 2011;33(8):638–42.
6. Steinert Y. Learning together: interprofessional education and faculty development. J Interprof Care. 2005;19(supp. 1):60–75.
7. Sandy LG, Bodenheimer T, Pawlson LG, Starfield B. The political economy of US primary care. Health Aff. 2009;28(4):1136–45.
8. Kelley MA, Connor A, Kun KE, Salmon ME. Social responsibility: conceptualization and embodiment in a school of nursing. Int J Nurs Educ Scholarsh. 2008;5:Article28.
9. Mullan F, Chen C, Petterson S, Kolsky G, Spagnola M. The social mission of medical education: ranking the schools. Ann Intern Med. 2010;152(12):804–11.
10. Vasilescu R, Barna C, Epure M, Baicu C. Developing university social responsibility: a model for the challenges of the new civil society. Proc Soc Behav Sci. 2010;2:4177–82.
11. Patrício M, Harden RM. The Bologna process—a global vision for the future of medical education. Med Teach. 2010;32(4):305–15.
12. Puschel K, Rojas P, Erazo A, Thompson B, Lopez J, Barros J. Social accountability of medical schools and academic primary care training in Latin America: principles but not practice. Fam Pract. 2014;31(4):399–408.
13. healthsocialaccountability.org. Global consensus for social accountability of medical schools [Internet]; 2010. http://healthsocialaccountability.org/. Accessed 29 Nov 2020.
14. Boelen C, Heck J. Defining and measuring the social accountability of medical schools. Geneva: World Health Organization; 1995. http://whqlibdoc.who.int/hq/1995/WHO_HRH_95.7.pdf. Accessed 29 Nov 2020.
15. Kwizera EN, Iputo JE. Addressing social responsibility in medical education: the African way. Med Teach. 2011;33(8):649–53.
16. National Ethical Guidelines for Biomedical and Health Research Involving Human Participants. New Delhi: Indian Council of Medical Research; 2017. http://icmr.nic.in/guidelines/ICMR_Ethical_Guidelines_2017.pdf

17. Ghoshal R. The social value of research: interrogating the paradoxes. Indian J Med Ethics. 2018;3(1):9–15.
18. Singh A, Anand A, Jaswal N. Implementing university/academicians' social responsibility conceptual framework in medical colleges. Ann Neurosci. 2019;26(3-4):8–9.
19. Rajput ASD. India aims for national policy on scientific social responsibility. Nature. 2019;574(7780):634.
20. Ramesh M. 'Scientific social responsibility' likely to be notified soon (2020). https://www.thehindubusinessline.com/news/science/scientific-social-responsibility-likely-to-be-notified-soon/article32796068.ece. Accessed 29 Nov 2020.
21. Anand A, Banik A, Minhas G, Bammidi S, Thakur K, Sharma K, et al. Creating a role model for "academicians" social responsibility (ASR) synergizing with Swachh Bharat Abhiyaan: a campus hygiene initiative by PGIMER, Chandigarh. Ann Neurosci. 2019;26(2):75–81.
22. Anand A. The case for academic social responsibility. Ann Neurosci. 2019;26(3-4):6–7.
23. Asif M, Searcy C. Towards a standardised management system for corporate sustainable development. TQM J. 2014;26(5).
24. Westcott RT. The certified manager of quality/organizational excellence handbook. 4th ed. ASQ Quality Management Division; 2013.
25. Hohnen P. Corporate social responsibility—an implementation guide for business; 2007. http://www.wame.org/resources/publication-ethics-policies-for-medical-journals/. Accessed 29 Nov 2020.
26. Kaushal S, Tyagi R, Banik A, Battu P, Mehra P, Sharma NK, Sharma K, Anand A. A unique data validation process by internal and external quality assurance system aimed to combat research malpractice. Int J Sci Res (IJSR). 2019;8(8):5–9.

12 Good Laboratory Practices: Lab Orientations, Meetings, and Value of Communication

Pooja Nadholta, Saras Jyoti, Sriloy Mohanty, Amit Singh, Jaideep Arya, and Neel Kamal Sharma

12.1 Introduction

A Research laboratory is a conventional form of vital and experiential learning, which is distinct from other forms of education. In general, research laboratories are controlled and regulated workplaces which provide facilities to conduct scientific research and experiments. A laboratory contains various sophisticated equipment, chemicals, and biomaterials that can be poisonous, flammable, explosive, radioactive, carcinogenic, and may require careful handling to minimize/ avoid injury and other associated health risks. The good laboratory practices must safeguard the health of research students working in the lab. Along with safety concerns, students who are working in the lab must know regarding the storage conditions/ procedure of usage and the place of storage of chemicals to work efficiently in the lab. Working in a place without having proper knowledge and understanding it becomes quite challenging and more time-consuming as compared to working in a familiar place. Therefore, to make things satisfying for the personnel working in a laboratory, it is essential to orient them about infrastructure, equipment, instruments, chemicals, and basic instructions of "how to use" and "how to handle." Seniors/ lab managers

P. Nadholta
Post Graduate Institute of Medical Education and Research, Chandigarh, India

S. Jyoti · J. Arya
Haryana Yog Council Ayush Department, Panchkula, Haryana, India

S. Mohanty
Center for Integrative Medicine and Research, AIIMS, New Delhi, India

A. Singh
Swami Vivekananda Yoga Anusandhana Samsansthana, Bangalore, Karnataka, India

N. K. Sharma (✉)
Noble Life Sciences Inc., Woodbine, MD, USA
e-mail: nsharma@noblelifesci.com

A. Anand (ed.), *Quality Assurance Implementation in Research Labs*,
https://doi.org/10.1007/978-981-16-3074-3_12

who are already working and managing the lab must share this with them. Besides lab orientations, communication, and time-to-time meetings among all the concerned persons, working, and organizing the laboratory are of supreme significance for improving the quality of research. To organize the laboratory and to make other research-related work more efficient, transparent, reproducible, and qualitative, some research laboratories implement Good Laboratory Practices (GLP) [1] and Standard Operating Procedures (SOPs) to ensure that all research activities are conducted efficiently and safely [2]. In a GLP system, it is essential to know and implement the quality management system, integrity, and reliability of the experiments.

Basically, GLP is an accepted method to conduct experiments and related operations in non-clinical laboratories ensuring the safety and quality of research work with efficient working in a regulated manner. It implies to the phrase "A little internal honesty" followed during research and helps in maintaining the records by documenting it for future reproducibility, transparency, and auditability. It not only includes the experimental part, but also defines the conditions and processes of organizations of how to plan, execute, monitor, record, and report the laboratory studies. GLP ensures that in a laboratory all the facilities are adequate, including well-maintained and timely calibrated equipment, jobs of individual personnel are well defined, and they are trained to do it, data is properly recorded, retained, and retrievable, all the documents, inventories, chemicals, instruments, and samples are properly labeled, handled, and stored in an organized manner. The GLP documents should be controlled, which means all the changes from the beginning till its archive should be maintained and kept properly [3]. Many new students who join the research laboratory are unfamiliar with this system of laboratory practices. They can be trained with periodic orientation, and their learning can be enhanced by encouraging them for discussions, interactions, meetings, and asking questions, which are an essential part of the research and development process.

12.2 Lab Orientations

Orientation is a process of orienting, introducing, and directing someone about where they are, what they are using, and how to use it in a proper manner. An easy example of orientation is training given to new employees or students when they first enter their new office, school, college, university, or research lab [4]. To start working in a new place with a new idea among new people, the prime thing is to know your workplace well with your responsibilities. Orientations give a holdup for newcomers with new information, experiences from those who already know, which helps in the academic success, personal growth of the newcomers and builds meaningful connections with others working at that place. Further, a well-planned orientation includes two-way communication, and Questions and Answers give an idea about expectations, potentials, mindsets, and interests of novices. The most important principle to convey during orientation is the commitment to improvement and continual learning by the team/supervisor.

Orientations to beginners must contain the following important points:

- Give a proper introduction of the person who is/are giving orientation.
- Make the beginners comfortable with the building/workplace/laboratory by giving a premises tour to introduce them to the facilities of the department.
- Introduce them nicely to colleagues/supervisors, and other coworkers.
- Briefly introduce them to the work of every person if necessary.
- Emphasize that they must follow their duties honestly, whenever assigned to them. Advise them to follow various checklists and procedures of the laboratory during enrollment, experiments, presentations, meetings, conferences, and writing.
- Adherence to the standard operating procedure increases consistency and uniformity.
- Point of contact should be clearly notified to the student at the time of orientation, so that they can approach the right person in case of any difficulty and confusion, e.g., when and which problem is to be discussed with which member of the Institute, department, and laboratory.
- Introduction to code and conduct, i.e., instruction sheets/rules of different practices, is necessary to get started with new work and workers at the new place.
- Safety and biomedical waste management procedures and policies should be described.
- Give them a chance to ask questions.
- Ask them to give their brief introduction, know their interests, ideas, and hobbies. Outlining the expectations for both the student and the supervisor is necessary to adhere to all standards.
- During orientation, keep asking them about their experience and take their inputs and suggestions for improving the next orientation and overall facilities.
- Ask them to share their feedback or overall experience.
- At the end of the orientation, tell them about the next topics that are necessary to orient them before starting work in the lab.

Topics of orientation can be:

- **Contact Information Orientation**: Names, contact numbers, and email addresses of colleagues, coworkers, supervisor, management, administration, safety, and security department should be provided.
- **Rights and Responsibility Orientation**: Every new person should be oriented about their rights and responsibilities towards work, the laboratory, and their duties.
- **Accident/Injury Reporting Procedures and Occupational Health**: Explain about the procedures to be followed in case of any injury or accident.
- **Emergency Procedures and Preparedness**: Contact info of emergency personnel, escaping plan, signals, sirens, and emergency exit routes, fire extinguishers, alarm pull boxes; location for eyewash in case of chemical spillage, fire, and gas leak should be explained.

- **Workplace Hazardous Material Information System (WHMIS)**: Explanation of the location, and proper labeling of hazardous substances/chemicals, hazardous symbols including the location and value of material safety data sheet (MSDS).
- **Personal Protective Equipment**: Importance of PPE, how and when to use it should be demonstrated to the students. PPE is anything that can protect you from direct contact with infectious agents, germs, and hazardous waste. It includes gloves, masks, shoe covers, head masks, gowns, etc. One must take precautions before handling infectious fluids, blood, touching waste material, and meeting any patient suffering from any kind of infection.
- **Hazardous Waste Removal**: Hazardous waste should be removed or disposed from time to time and should not be stored for a longer period. This information should be clear to every individual, and they should know about the associated risks.
- **Biosafety and Chemical Safety**: MSDS contains information on all the hazards associated with chemicals. Labeling of all the chemicals and its contents and associated hazards should be done properly and explained to every person of the lab. Below (Fig. 12.1) is the attached format of rules and regulations to be followed for chemical inventories.
- **Fire Safety**: Orientation regarding fire safety management and the use of fire extinguishers with a practical demonstration should be given. In laboratories, special care should also be taken while keeping the flammable chemicals. These are generally labeled red with a flammable sticker. These chemicals should always be stored in a flammable **chemical** cabinet.
- A log register for electrical items like refrigerators, ACs is good to maintain to avoid any failure and fire. Everyone in the laboratory must be aware of the nearest fire alarm pull station, exit doors, evacuation plan, and Institute fire control department numbers.
- Following precautions should be taken into consideration while working in the laboratory:
  - Before operating any instrument, go through the manual once and be familiar with its controls and features.
  - Operate the instrument as per the manufacturer's instructions.
  - Turn off the equipment after using and when not in use.
  - Before leaving the laboratory, duly check the equipment, ACs, refrigerators, and switches.
  - Do not keep flammable liquids near heat-producing equipment, flashpoints, and refrigerators (which are not suitable for storing flammable liquids).
  - Avoid extension cords, and if using them, do not make the cluster of wires.
  - Make different cabinets and refrigerators for flammable liquids and clearly label them.

A format for research laboratory safety orientation is provided (Fig. 12.2).

Record-Keeping Orientation about the importance of record archiving and different ways to keep the records should be given. Students must be aware of the process

Rules, regulations, procedures and precautions of the lab and workstation where chemicals are used or stored:

- Place and use procedure for hand wash and eye-wash area
- Place and use procedure for all fire extinguishers (DO NOT use if you don't know how)
- Place and use procedure of emergency showers
- Place and use procedure of emergency contacts (phone numbers)
- Place and use procedure of First Aid Kits along with contents (keep regular check for expiry date of medicine)
- Place for getting access card/keys
- Procedure and immediately notify (concerned authority) for reporting of lab accidents and near-misses
- Place and list of Chemical Safety Manual (both Soft copy and Hard copy)
- Place of spill kits, when and how to use them, whom to contact
- Place and use procedure of MSDS, how to use them
- Maintenance of catalogue and steps for ordering chemicals, supplies, instruments/equipment, cylinders
- Chemical Barcodes
- Place and use procedure of emergency alarms- fire, fume hood air flow, emergency notification system, other equipment-specific alarms
- Precautions and procedure of maintaining the Fume hoods
- Labeling of workplace/workstation
- Records and procedure of maintaining Gas Cylinders - transferring/moving, storage precautions, health hazards and how to return (if rental)
- Use procedure and precautions of maintaining the liquid nitrogen dewars, frost, cryogenic hazards
- Precautions and health hazards of harmful reactive compounds, peroxides, oxidizers, toxic materials, corrosives, and amines
- Use procedure of labeling storing and weighing of chemicals
- Notify the concerned lab authority for expired chemicals
- Use and transporting of bottles & location of carriers
- Use procedure and proper storage/use of flammables, acids, bases, etc.
- Labeling of Fridges
- Procedure to dispose of broken glass/sharp containers/flask
- Contact information for experiments involving harmful/hazardous chemicals (especially when working alone)
- Understanding of general wet lab safety rules - location and contents
  - Use of safety glasses along with storage locations,
  - Use Procedure of washing solution

Fig. 12.1 Rules, regulation, procedures, and precautions for chemical inventories

and benefits of keeping a record of everything they do. The record management system ensures compliance, improves efficiency and traceability of data. All the members of the lab get complete access to the same information when needed, which decreases the chances of non-verbal communication. Good record management cuts the costs and saves the time and efforts that one may invest to store, print, and find once lost. Formats of an academic log sheet (Fig. 12.3) is shown, which can be used in a laboratory for ensuring compliance to GLP and to keep a proper record of chemical or other lab resources used while working in a lab.

Research laboratory Safety Orientation

I ______________________________ working in the capacity of ______________________________ under the supervision of ______________________________ , fully understand the following Safety Orientation given by ______________________________

Following points should be covered during laboratory safety orientation:

- No eating/drinking/smoking/gum in lab - consumption or storage as well
- Avoid Cosmetic application in lab
- Washing of hands at designated washing area
- Lab coat should not be worn outside the lab
- Use procedure of Gloves – when to use, and how to dispose
- No earphones in lab
- Avoid wearing loose/shorts clothes in lab
- Avoid wearing jewelry
- Never smell or taste chemicals.
- Do not pipette by mouth.
- Avoid carrying Mobile phone to workstation/Fume hoods
- Wear only closed toe covered shoes in labs
- Use procedure of personal protective equipment kits
- Use procedures of respirators (needs proper training)
- Security/safety – Do's/Don'ts
- Lab managers should ensure contractors/visitors must follow safety rules while entering into labs
- Hazards of using equipment -Electrical hazards/Cord fitting
- Use procedure and precautions to be taken while working with radiation and laser
- Lab committee for prevention of harassment, discrimination, violence and bullying, inequality
- Policy for working alone/or during holidays
- Monthly safety inspections and Feedback /reports
- Housekeeping standards
- Use of lab Computer/Phone:
- Role of lab managers/Seniors
- Consequences for non-compliance or mismanagement

Signature of PI ______________ Presenter's Signature ______________________

Date ______________________ Date ______________________________

Fig. 12.2 Format for research laboratory safety orientation

Academic log sheet

Student name________________ **Position______________**

Supervisor's name____________ **Year__________________**

Academic log sheet contains the annual activities of students and PI assess the academic progress of student annually by checking academic log sheet.

Sr.no.	Academic activity	Attended	Signature of PI
1.	Discussions	30	
2.	Lab meeting	40	
3.	Journal club	70	
4.	Seminars	12	
5.	Conferences	5	
6.	Workshops	7	
7.	Genetic meeting	6	
8.	Animal meeting	6	
9.	Quality assurance meeting	5	
10.	Leaves	15	
11.	DC meetings	2	
12.	Orientation	8	

Fig. 12.3 Format of the academic log sheet

These are some very basic and important points, which should be introduced to a new person.

Introductory orientation is the beginning of the process of making beginners familiar to a new place/work. The cascade of orientation must flow throughout the journey until novices reach the expert state. A format checklist that can be followed for beginner's orientation is shown (Fig. 12.4).

Orientation checklist

Student name: ____________________ Supervisor's name: ____________________

Joining date: ____________________ Location: ____________________

INSTRUCTIONS:

This form will be used to document student's participation in different orientations listed below. As each orientation is completed, both student and instructor will sign in the appropriate box and date of orientation completion will be mentioned in box. When form will be complete, student will be given a certificate of orientation completion.

S. No.	Topics	Student's initial	Instructor's initial	Date
1.	Basic introduction orientation.			
2.	GLP orientation			
3.	First aid orientation			
4.	Contact information orientation.			
5.	Rights and Responsibility orientation.			
6.	Accident/Injury Reporting Procedures and Occupational Health.			
7.	Emergency Procedures and Preparedness.			
8.	Workplace Hazardous Material Information System (WHMIS).			
9.	Biosafety and Chemical Safety.			
10.	Hazardous Waste Removal.			
11.	Personal Protective Equipment.			
12.	Fire safety.			
13.	Animal orientation			
14.	Quality Assurance Orientation			
15.	Record keeping.			

Fig. 12.4 Orientation checklist format

12.3 Different Models of Skill Acquisition

Any beginner, who wants to excel in a particular subject, could either flounder with trial-and-error method or seek aid from an expert. When it comes to laboratory experiments, it is always the second method that is safe and productive. A skill acquisition model describes how learners gain new skills by passing through many orientations, communication, meetings, and discussions. In 1980, two brothers, Stuart and Hubert Dreyfus, proposed the first model of skill acquisition in the field of education and operations research. This model suggested that students pass through five distinct stages of adroitness which are: (1) novice, (2) competence, (3) proficiency, (4) expertise, and (5) mastery. Each stage is a successive transformation of the student resulting in making him/her more intuitive and automated.

Another important point to note is that it is essential for both the learner and the trainer/demonstrator to understand the stages of skill development. A detailed understanding of skill acquisition stages is essential for the development of an effective and impactful training/ orientation.

Below is the brief introduction of each stage given by Stuart and Hubert Dreyfus [5]:

Stage 1: Novice

This stage of skill acquisition requires no previous experiential background or understanding of the laboratory situation. The educator or instructors should provide detailed step-wise instructions to accomplish a task to the novice under personal observation. The student is coached to follow the SOPs strictly. Novices have very limited knowledge to forecast the forthcoming situation, so the limitations and contraindications should be explained in length. It is observed that instructional feedback techniques are useful in improving the understanding of the student.

Stage 2: Competence

This is the second stage of the skill acquisition method, which comes with considerable experience, where the student is no more dependent on the instructions of the expert and has a productive pattern of working. This stage builds a new level of responsibility and comfort in the student at the laboratory, resulting in heightened experiential learning. An expert should incorporate different methods to make the student calm and composed during the experiments as the students in this stage generally rely on the SOPs and may have difficulty recognizing the variations in the outcomes of experiments.

Stage 3: Proficiency

Repeated practice of the experiments exposes the student to a wide range of variations in the outcomes. At this stage, the student knows how to deal with the situation when it is not going according to the SOPs. This stage enables the student to develop a greater sense of salience. In this state, the student needs to understand and respect the work of the colleagues, and at the same time, continue to learn more from the colleagues and experts.

Stage 4: Expertise

This stage is the transitional stage on the way to mastery on the field. After gathering knowledge and experience from many situations, now the student reacts intuitively and appropriately to the situation by not only performing the task but also controlling it. The previous stages were quantitatively increasing the capability of the performance, whereas now the student makes qualitative improvement in the way he/she performs in a demanding situation.

Stage 5: Mastery

Although expertise is the highest level of the mental improvement process, but mastery is the state when an expert can consciously put all their energy/experience/expertise into the performance. He/she no longer has to put effort into the process of his performance, can effortlessly perform the appropriate action as per the demand of the situation. Intuitive links develop between seeing and responding to the situation in the laboratory. This is the stage where he/she can share their knowledge with the novice.

There are two more steps that were not found originally in the report of Stuart and Hubert Dreyfus but are pivotal in good research practice.

Stage 6: Decision

This stage is an extension of mastery in which the student has now mastered the techniques after an experience of years. The expert can now take decisions regarding the tests and, while guiding the student, is no more in need of taking help from the seniors or experts like before.

Stage 7: Awareness

At this point, the student can take precise decisions and perform as if it is their second nature. At this stage, the students are allowed to guide their juniors and help them improve their skills.

12.4 Communication

Communication domain is a social sphere to subvert the existing standard, and bring in new, more productive standards by combining the inputs from interaction among diverse minds and become the driver of change to accommodate a new proposition [6]. Communication is not only a realization of one's own actions, but it also gives a person new ways to execute plan of actions, if previous one is not working. Communication can be verbal or written, formal or informal, and with professionals or colleagues. Each kind of communication adds to the existing skills and its implications in a right manner. Communication among all the individuals involved in a particular study is of paramount importance to plan the study effectively, to address problems during the study, and to execute the plan as scheduled. Many problems associated with studies can be prevented and resolved by effective communication among concerned persons involved in that particular study [7].

For multi-site studies, as well as in a laboratory, where students are helping each other in their work, it is imperative for everyone to know about their responsibilities and the status of others' work. Lack and delay in communication can significantly harm both the student and investigator, which can further contribute to compromised quality as well as lead to an impeded schedule and hence results.

Despite verbal communication being considered as the preferred procedure for discussions, sharing ideas, and troubleshooting problems, newly emerging non-verbal means of communication, are now more acceptable because it is an easy and not time-bound.

12.5 Activities to Improve Communication Skills

The main importance of communication skills is to develop communique capability in prospective researchers so that they can transfer thoughts, information, and ideas with precision and clarity. The activities mentioned below will improve a student's communication skills with an emphasis on taming their oral communiqué, both in informal and formal situations:

1. **Writing and Reading Activities**: Reading, writing, speaking, and listening activities should be encouraged among students for their overall development [8]. Consistent reading not only improves writing skills but also helps in perfecting oratory skills. Reading is a key component for improving both written and spoken communication. According to the famous essayist Francis Bacon, among the four skills listening, speaking, reading, and writing–reading is the most pivotal skill because a reader can rebel the pitfall of listening, speaking, and writing in terms of language and understanding. A good reader is always a good communicator, and every student is advised to gain good reading skills at the earliest [9].
2. **Discussion Activities**: Every type of discussion is vital for the progress of both, the student and the project. Regular productive discussions with PI, colleagues, and coworkers keep the students focused and directed at their work. It is suggested to make a discussion roster of every person in the laboratory, once or twice in a week, where the student can discuss about his/her problems, progress, ideas, and hurdles that they are facing with the PI. Along with this, they can also show their records, results, log sheets, and logbooks to the PI so that the PI can ensure GLP adherence by students in the laboratory. Regular discussion builds confidence and improves the skills of the students, and upgrades their way of thinking, which can prevent them from misunderstanding things in the future and excel in their field of work. The template SOP that can be followed for discussion day is given (Fig. 12.5).
3. **Making an Effective Power Point Presentation**: Presentation skills are much needed to deliver an effective and engaging presentation. Presentation skills include the presentation structure, design of slides, body language, good/formal dress up and voice tone. Below are some tips to make your slides effective:

STANDARD OPERATING PROCEDURE

<table>
<tr><td colspan="5">Title: Discussion Day</td></tr>
<tr><td>SOP No.</td><td>Edition No.</td><td>Effective Date</td><td>Review Date</td><td rowspan="2">Document Controller
(Signature/Stamp)</td></tr>
<tr><td>Copy No.</td><td>Date of Issue</td><td colspan="2">Location (Unit/Division)</td></tr>
</table>

Principle:-

1. Discussion with Study Director/PI are as important as attending and presenting Seminars, journal clubs as well as attending lab meetings. In the absence of formal PhD curriculum, these academic activities add value to research activities and sustain productivity. The lab meetings provide a vibrant platform to discuss individual progress, difficulties and other problems and ideas in carrying out investigations.

2. Status: Original ☐ Amended☐ Revised☐ Revalidated ☐

3. Approvals:

	Name	Signature	Date
Author			
Q.A. Review			
Study Director			

Fig. 12.5 Standard operating protocol for discussion day

(a) Effective slides are the robust module of a successful presentation, so *"do your slides right or do not do it at all"* [10].
(b) Before making a PowerPoint presentation, prepare a story that you want to tell to your audience.
(c) Remove the unnecessary part of the presentation.
(d) Instead of sentences, lace up it with images, schematics, and structures.

(e) Make your presentation short and precise.
(f) In the end, give a clear and precise conclusion and a take away message.

4. **Attending and Understanding Activities**: Just like swimming cannot be learnt just by reading and observing, in the same way, communication skills cannot be developed just by reading, writing, listening, and observing. Constant practice is necessary to develop good communication skills, but before practicing, one must know what to practice. To get started with the development of communication skills, start attending the events and understand them. Students can follow below-mentioned activities:

   (a) Attend orientations and other events when they join a new Institute.
   (b) Interact with colleagues and coworkers.
   (c) Actively attend discussions, lab meetings, and orientations.
   (d) Attend academic activities of the Institute, such as Journal clubs, seminars, and other presentations.
   (e) Deliver presentations and prepare for it by practicing more

5. **Making a Speech**: Choose a topic and a person in front of whom you do not hesitate to speak and give a speech on your chosen topic. It prepares you for other formal discussions, presentations, and speeches.
6. **Group Discussion participation**: Do not hesitate to put your point of view in any discussion. Active participation not only helps in generating new ideas, but also helps in upgrading knowledge, overall growth and makes discussions more productive.
7. **Oral Presentation**: Oral presentation refers to delivering your thoughts on a specific topic live, in front of an audience. A well-planned and rehearsed presentation gathers the audience's attention and makes it easy for them to understand the message that you want to convey.
8. **Mock Interviews**: A practice job interview, which is being held with a professional, is known as a mock interview. A Mock interview develops an enhanced confidence and interview skills [11] .

12.6 Naming and Categorization of a Communication Medium

Communication is the act of exchanging information from one person, organization, place, or group to another by speaking, writing, showing signs, symbols, pictures, and videos. Etymological meaning of the term "communication" is sharing or distributing [12] .

12.6.1 Types of Communication

Mainly communication can be divided into verbal, non-verbal, visual, and written communication.

- Verbal communication is a form of communication in which the information is conveyed verbally by speaking to someone. The efficiency by which it is understood depends upon the language in which the message is conveyed. In multilinguistic laboratories, verbal communication is less efficient.
- Non-verbal communication is a non-linguistic representation of information. It includes body language, gestures, facial expression, and other behavioral clues. This medium of communication is less efficient because it contains comparatively less or unclear information, and what is being conveyed may not be received in the same way by the receiver [13] .
- Written communication refers to sending information in a written form through letters, emails, WhatsApp, text messages, master schedules, and log sheets. It is an efficient and formal way to put your point clearly
- Visual communication involves the idea of conveying messages/information through a visible medium in the form of pictures, videos, graphs, designs, and drawings [14] .

Monthly Submission of Master Schedules

Master schedule (MS) is a schedule built in anticipation for planning the work to be done till a specific upcoming date. Usually, a 1-month work plan is scheduled by the student with a target date of accomplishment and is sent to the study director for further modification. It includes the list of assignments, projects, and other commitments. Master schedule is usually sent for a period of month, and compliance is assessed by lab meetings and discussions [15] .

MS of the upcoming month should be sent to the study director/PI at the end of the previous month. It not only puts your preferences in the notice of the PI, but also helps the PI to manage his time for meetings and discussions regarding the work schedule. MS also helps the students to accomplish the work in an organized and timely manner. The format that can be used to make and adhere to a monthly MS is shown (Fig. 12.6).

12.6.2 Categorization of Communication

Communication, i.e., exchange of information, ideas, and thoughts can be done in different ways as described above. Every communication between different people has a different significance, value, and outcome. We categorize communication and its importance with different individuals/committees/groups as below:

12.6.2.1 PI and Student

Experience can make complex things easier and more interesting to do. For the execution of a plan and then ensuring consistency, PI plays a leading role. The student/research scholar can give a better output if they are directed on the right path by productive inputs/ideas and proper guidance. As the project progresses, the next step comes with a new milestone, and the level of difficulties also increase. If not

Master schedule

Month__________________________

Name of student____________________

Name of PI________________________

Week	Activities	Done (Please tick)	If not (Reason)	Signature of student	Signature of PI
1ST Week	➢ Activity 1 ➢ Activity 2 ➢ Activity 3 ➢ Activity 4				
2nd Week	➢ Activity 1 ➢ Activity 2 ➢ Activity 3 ➢ Activity 4 ➢ Activity 5				
3rd Week	➢ Activity 1 ➢ Activity 2 ➢ Activity3				
4th Week	➢ Activity 1 ➢ Activity 2 ➢ Activity 3				

Fig. 12.6 Monthly master schedule format

given proper guidance and encouragement, disappointments can dominate the vision to achieve the goal. Discussing the problems with the PI can be the easiest and most efficient way to keep students motivated and to give work a new pace. Therefore, it is recommended to never break a communication thread with the PI for better progress and to work efficiently.

12.6.2.2 PI and QA

Quality Assurance (QA) assures the GLP adherence, student's progress, laboratory's condition, availability of lab resources, inventories, proper use of chemicals before they expire, daily/weekly investigation of instruments, and quality. QA is a way to impede the mistakes and enhance the quality, hence improving progress and outcomes. Discussion/communication between PI and QA person is foremost to ensure the quality and fulfill the requirements to maintain the quality of work in a lab.

12.6.2.3 Student and Doctoral Committee

In research Institutes, Doctoral committee (DC) consists of a group of experts chosen by the Institute to give suggestions related to students' projects, to analyze the progress, pace of work, scope of doing work, and orient the students in the right direction. Because periodic DC meetings play an important role in strategizing, implementing, and executing the project, the following points should be followed before organizing a meeting:

- Visit every member with a copy of your project and ask them for their available three dates for meetings.
- Take email IDs and contact numbers of every DC member.
- Keep the meeting on a date when every member is available.
- Make a notice and get it signed by every member before the meeting date.
- Send them a reminder, the venue (meeting link in case of an online meeting) one day before the meeting.
- Prepare your presentation well and rehearse in the lab before the meeting.
- Discuss your final slides with the PI before the final presentation.
- Take suggestions from every member and work on them.

12.6.2.4 Student and Student

Learning is the byproduct of a conversation. Whether the conversation is with self, internal or external dialogs, or something that we read, listen, observe, interpret, or analyze—we always learn something [16]. Hearing someone else's thoughts on any idea increases the understanding, memory, and observation of one's own thinking. Informal, oral, and friendly conversations among students where their thoughts are not monitored by anyone else help in refining and solidifying their thoughts.

Informal communications between lab mates over lunch or tea create a strong bonding between them. These communications may involve discussions over movies/ series, a healthy lifestyle, new restaurants, or news, etc. This refreshes the mind and body. Laughter during these hours transforms the whole scenario in the lab.

12.6.2.5 Junior and Senior Student

Senior students are always a storehouse of knowledge, experience, and ideas. Learning from the experiences of seniors can make things easier and less time-consuming. Seniors guide Junior students throughout their journey for sustainable growth and development.

12.7 Value of Communication

Communication at the workplace refines the goals and helps the whole team, including coworkers, and helps in collaboration in order to work in a systematic way. This fundamental practice/skill establishes a fruitful workforce that can effectively encourage team members to work and produce results. Different mediums and categories of communication that are described in this chapter can help in achieving a goal in a much faster, easier, and productive manner. Effective communication at the workplace offers several benefits:

- Positive engagement to work
- Keeps the focus on the goal
- Shared ideas and efforts
- Proper guidance

- Troubleshooting
- Increases the pace of work
- Proper planning and execution.

Confidentiality of Communication and Orientations "Privileged conversation" is delivered by one individual to another, without the involvement of a third person before, during and after the conversation except when a third person is required as the interpreter of language. Privileged conversations are confidential and build trust between the speaker and the listener. The principle of confidentiality is about privacy and respect. For a team to work together and grow together, maintaining confidentiality is a prime factor followed in GLP.

Is Language a Barrier in Communication?
Language is a fundamental method of human communication, consisting of different words combined in a standard and organized manner conveyed by speaking, writing, and using different gestures. Different countries and even different parts of the same country have different languages that residents use to communicate with each other. The difficulties experienced in communication by people from different regions who speak different languages are known as a linguistic barrier or a language barrier. It becomes difficult to communicate when multi-ethnic and multinational students/employees work in the same place. Students struggle to express and communicate when working in a laboratory where the students' first language is not used as a communication language. This can also impact the mental health of the student and affect their propensity to learn. According to Wittgenstein, "The limits of our language" means the limits of our world [17]. In this situation, no-verbal and visual communication can act as an adjuvant to help the students adjust and learn.

To overcome the language barrier, PI should ensure that the communication should be in plain language, use visual method of communication, repeat the sentence, provide classes to students and be respectful. It can be challenging, but working with persons from different backgrounds leads to innovation, success, and creativeness.

12.8 Lab Meetings

In the twenty-first century, where it is convenient to communicate over mails or phone, most of the laboratories across the world still conduct standard laboratory meetings. These meetings not only establish and cultivate a laboratory culture but also foster a sense of community in the laboratory. Lab meetings are also a platform to discuss the progress, pitfalls, problem-solving, and collaborative efforts. Many laboratories still follow formal laboratory meetings with one presenter, with a slide highlighting the overview, current updates, problems faced, and possible strategies to overcome the problems. Though these meetings serve as orientation meetings for the freshers in the laboratory, others may find it to be monotonous and lengthier. Many laboratories now-a-days are opting for a more informal meeting, where the student brings his lab notes and images and discusses the same with the team without a slide. This technique makes it less intimidating for the presenter and more convenient for other members as it reduces the meeting time. Either ways, the student gains exposure to new research questions, theories, methodologies, and understanding of the unique strengths of the colleagues in the lab.

Laboratory meetings can be either individual meetings or team meetings. Each meeting has its own advantages and disadvantages. Individual meetings are generally short in duration and are mostly target-oriented based on weekly reports. The main aim of these meetings is to address the immediate concerns and allow the flow of work without any hindrance. Other members of the lab may not be familiar with the project, and as a result, the student may feel isolated in their project. On the other hand, group meetings are difficult to schedule as it requires everyone in the laboratory to attend them. Moreover, for many senior lab members, these become monotonous as mentioned above, while junior members look forward to these as means to learn and communicate. There are a few other categories of meetings, which will be discussed further.

Laboratories generally have their monthly master schedules, including group meetings, presentations, Journal club presentations, abstract, and poster sessions. Individual meetings are often not listed in the master schedule and are done to address immediate challenges in the lab.

12.8.1 Meetings Matter-Effects of Team Meetings on Team and Organizational Success

Team meetings are indispensable as they promote the success of the team members as well as the organization. During meetings, the expertise of individual team members can help in the development of new ideas, new protocols, new decisions, and suggestions which can change the process and can increase the progress rate. Regular meetings to discuss the progress, hurdles, work reports, and shortcomings can be organized in each laboratory to tap the potential and to enhance the efficacy of work and hence, the output. As suggested by Liker and Meier, meetings and discussions are the vitals of continuous progress. Knowledge of one person can be used for the growth of another person and vice-versa [18, 19]. There is a lot of difference between planning and executing, as these processes may be influenced by the availability of resources, guidelines, support, and many other factors. To streamline the execution and planning, communication acts as a bridge between the project investigator and the manager (usually research fellow, project assistant, research associate). Throughout the implementation stage, the knowledge level of both, the project investigator and research fellow changes over time as the work progresses. If both of them do not discuss about the changes, progress, and limitations, it becomes difficult or challenging to further continue and complete the project at the scheduled time points. In a similar manner, these communications can be turned into discussions and meetings with more experienced persons, as persons who are involved in the project may not have enough knowledge or ideas to continue with the work, and the other panel can give a better insight towards the same plan [20] . Time-to-time meetings (weekly meetings) build morale, identify small problems before they become large, identify good ideas earlier rather than later, share information and training with all the staff, communicate key issues and try to find solutions for them.

A key part of meeting is making "meeting minutes." Minutes, also known as notes, are instant written records of a meeting, which typically describes the events and discussions of meetings along with the list of attendees, absentees, statements of each individual regarding their work, statement of the issue being considered, and related responses or decisions for the issue. Each minute (note) is intended to remind the readers of a decision that was reached and actions that should be taken as a consequence. The main purpose of minutes is to provide a public memory for a group and to assess their successive growth and record problems and progress alike. The standard operating procedure (SOP) for conducting lab meetings for assessing the progress of researchers in the laboratory and for planning the further progress of work is given (Fig. 12.7). This SOP is being used in Neuroscience Research Lab, PGIMER, Chandigarh.

12.8.2 How to Run a Successful Meeting

For a successful meeting following points should be considered before starting a meeting:

1. **Scheduling a Lab Meeting**
   Generally, lab meetings are weekly. However, it can be tailored as per the need, workflow, and lab experiments. The PI may have a rigid schedule on a particular day and time, or it can be fixed as per the convenience of the team. It is advised to keep meetings at a particular time of the week or month as per the need.
2. **Duration of the Meeting**
   One to one and a half hour seems to be an average lab meeting time, although some meetings may last upto 3 h depending on number of students. The first 15 min are to review the decisions and implications of the last meeting, the next 30–45 min are to review the data and updates of the project, followed by 15 min of brainstorming over the possible solutions. Generally, most of the decisions are taken at the final minutes of the lab meetings. It is always advised to keep the meeting shorter.
3. **Agenda of the Meeting**
   Setting up an agenda is a work of dexterity, keeping realistic goals and the time allotted for the meetings. The meeting agenda should be circulated prior to the meeting to all the members attending, not only to give direction to the meeting but also for setting expectations for the members attending the meeting. The agenda should accompany the materials to be discussed. For example, if it is a paper presentation or a Journal club, the paper to be discussed shall be shared with the attendees prior to the meeting. The agenda should also assign roles to the attendees, including a moderator, a presenter, a timekeeper, and a note-taker. This helps in making the most out of meetings in a more efficient way.

STANDARD OPERATING PROCEDURE

Title: Lab meeting				
SOP No.	**Edition No.**	**Effective Date**	**Review Date**	**Document Controller** **(Signature/Stamp)**
Copy No.	**Date of Issue**	**Location (Unit/Division)**		

1. Lab meetings are held every week at specific day and specific time at workplace or digitally where concerned persons can join the meeting. Attendance of each concerned personnel is mandatory to make meeting effective. It may last up to 3-4 hrs and intended to summarize the output of past week and plan for the forthcoming week.
2. In every lab meeting one 'theme presentation' is done where bulk of talk is done by the research personnel.
3. Important announcements, suggestions etc are discussed in such meetings.

4. Status: **Original** ☐ **Amended** ☐ **Revised** ☐ **Revalidated** ☐

5. Approvals:

	Name	**Signature**	**Date**
Author			
Q.A. Review			
Review by Study Director			
Management Approval			

Fig. 12.7 Standard operating procedure for lab meeting

4. **During the Meeting**

   In lab meetings, time management should be given a high priority as most of the attendees might have come to participate, keeping their work aside. The meeting should start and continue as per the pre set agenda and end in time. The seniors or the PI should keep a track on the flow of the discussion and try to keep it focused in order to arrive at a conclusion. Everyone should participate in the final discussion.

5. **Summarizing and Sharing the Minutes**

   After the discussions and the decisions, the PI or senior lab members should summarize the discussions, decisions, and future implementations. The presenter may then make a "minute of the meeting" and circulate the same after getting it checked by the PI. Sample draft of the meeting is attached below (Fig. 12.8).

a

Restricted Circulation **Photocopying Prohibited**

Title: Lab Meeting Minutes (Date)			
Edition No.	Effective Date	Review Date	Document Controller (Signature/Stamp)
Date of Issue	Location (Unit/Division)		

Summary

Meeting was convened by Supervisor (Name) at (Time) AM on (Date) at (Place). Following is the discussion among the research scholars and Supervisor. The list of those who attended the meeting has reproduced below. Meeting minutes are:

Student 1 informed that he is writing thesis paper. She done RNA isolation, FACS and RTPCR and planning to do ELISA next week. Along with this she will write manuscript and will review.

Student 2 informed that she is writing review and working on another paper. She also told about her next week plan.

Student 3 informed that she will submit manuscript of Correlation b/w different biomarkers in targeted journal till Monday and this has to be reminded to supervisor in next lab meeting.

Supervisor advised everyone to follow master schedule, complete assigned work on time, ask for resources if needed, inform about advance leaves, report on time, continue compliance to GLP and attend daily discussions.

Attended by:

1. **Student 1**
2. **Student 2**
3. **Student 3**
4. **Student 4**

Absentees:

1. **Student 9**
2. **Student 10**

Approvals:	Name	Signature	Date
Prepared By			
Q.A. Review			
Approved By Study Director			

PGIMER HR09 **Neuroscience Research Lab**

Fig. 12.8 (**a**, **b**) Formats for making lab meeting minutes

b

XYZ Research Lab – Meeting Minutes Format

Objective-

Date- DD-MMM-YYYY **Time-00:00:00**

Meeting Facilitator-

Name	Attendees	Excused
A	X	
B	X	
C	X	
D	X	
E	X	

Agenda

1-
2-
3-

Insights/Feedback

1-
2-
3-

Question & Answer

1-
2-
3-

Fig. 12.8 (continued)

6. **Follow-Up of the Implementation**
   The decisions taken in the meeting should be followed for smooth functioning of the laboratory and should be reviewed periodically by the senior members and PI. The same also can be discussed in the first 10 min of the next meeting.

12.8.3 How to Make the Most Out of a Lab Meeting

The lab meetings can help students in skill acquisition and widen their knowledge by introducing new theories and methodologies. The student should follow 3 P's to make the most out of these as below

1. **Prepare for the Meeting**
   The student should go through the agenda and the materials shared for the meeting and accordingly read the background of the study, recent research papers and articles. He/she should make a list of questions and additional information regarding the topic. If given the role of a moderate or a note-taker, the student should also be prepared for the same.
2. **Participate in the Discussions**
   The student should try to make the most out of the meeting by participating in the discussions, asking questions, sharing their knowledge based on the preparation done prior to the meetings. A healthy discussion regarding the topic being discussed is always rewarding. He/she should always try to contribute to the meeting, instead of just sitting and observing.
3. **Present or Moderate a Meeting**
   Presenting in laboratory meetings gives a platform to gain confidence for presenting in workshops and conferences. Moderating a meeting also requires a lot of preparation and understanding of the subject. The more a student takes these roles, the stronger his/her public speaking qualities become.

12.8.4 Importance of Lab Meetings

The purpose of lab meetings is to establish a lab culture that infuses accountability to lab activities and share new ideas. It is a good platform to practice communication skills, enhance decision making and problem-solving besides maximizing the success of all projects together, sharpen critical thinking, and to celebrate the achievements of the lab. Lab meetings play a key role in developing enthusiasm, working spirit, new ideas, and new knowledge not only in the students' particular fields, but also in the relative fields in which other students are working. In meetings students should not hesitate to ask anytime, "I did not understand it, can you please explain again?".

Problem-solving interaction and action planning are significantly more satisfactory when discussed with the other members and especially with the expert in that particular field in their meetings. Better meetings are associated with a higher team productivity, hence greater results, and better efficiency. Therefore, regular meetings and discussions shape both the team and the organizational outcomes by adding more value to the quality of work [21]. During the meetings, students self-evaluate themselves and also evaluate the other person (in case of a one-to-one meeting) or persons (in case of group meetings) on the basis of previous meeting minutes.

12.9 Challenges and Opportunities in Operationalizing Periodic Lab Communication Activities

Problems of communication are quite common in multinational and multi-lingual international labs, especially when students or workers come from different regions with different nationalities and have different training, qualifications, or knowledge levels. Operationalizing GLP and its vital component—communication, becomes a hurdle and a matter of concern in such laboratories due to the above-mentioned factors, and these hurdles are further compounded as GLP is not widely practiced in other laboratories. Even in the laboratories which do not follow GLP regulations, these hurdles can be overcome by implementing scheduled, formal, informal meetings, orientations, and discussions within and without laboratories and also between the principal investigator and the research fellows. In addition to these hurdles, dysfunctional communication such as complaining, criticizing others, and tattling impart a negative effect on growth and act as an adjuvant for further barricades in progress, which should be avoided.

12.10 Interactions That Help in Training the Students to Practice Their Skills

12.10.1 Formal Presentations

A presentation represents how we perceive and process the information. Presentations give new students an opportunity to receive suggestions and new insights. Presenting data clearly and efficiently sometimes becomes quite challenging for students. We discuss some essential points for effectively presenting the data. The presentation should be understandable and well-structured and should be delivered in the given time slot.

Every presentation should start with a title page containing the name of the topic, the presenter's name as well as the date on which the presentation has been given. Headers and footers should be included as appropriate. The presented information should focus on the main agenda and should be presented point by point rather than in a paragraph. The presentation should include images and flow charts for ease of understanding. The presentation should focus on and cover major areas related to methodology, results, discussions (can include result gaps, ongoing clinical trials (If any), successful clinical trials, If any, and conclusion. Other data such as calculations and raw data should be presented in the back-up slides (shown when requested). The use of study-related audios and videos in the presentation makes up for better understanding. For the sake of improving the quality, peers, and the supervisor should review the final presentation, and the comments should be addressed appropriately before sharing the presentation with the attendees. The pre-knowledge, present scenario and the foreseen outcomes should also be clear from the presentation.

12.10.2 Abstract/Poster Session

An Abstract and Poster session is the best way to represent your work and yourself to the peer scientists and leaders. The visual presentation should include only relevant and organized text, fine pictorial quality pictures, and a clear background. The visual impact of the poster should be imperishable.

The information should be presented in a fluent, clear, and rhythmic manner. The information flow should be logical and facilitate interpretation. During the presentation, the use of gestures by the speaker plays a pivotal role in engaging the listeners and should be used as often as possible. Presentations during conferences can be rehearsed in front of the lab mates in order to feel more confident and to overcome nervousness. Group discussions and constructive criticism always improve the performance of the students. A successful presentation requires collaboration and inputs shared by the teammates. The unique ideas exchanged between labmates can encourage brainstorming.

12.10.3 Journal Clubs

In order to keep one's knowledge updated, the role of Journals clubs is of immense importance. The publications based on recent researches in various parts of the world should be discussed. It will encourage the new students to lay a firm foot in presenting their own innovations and researches to the other colleagues in the lab. It will not only help in implementing new ideas, but will encourage others to achieve more.

12.10.4 Progress Update

For continuous performance and, eventually, success, the "4A" rule can be followed, which is :

1. Action
2. Activity
3. Accomplishment
4. Advancement

The weekly report must include the "4A" rule as a weekly planner. The real-time weekly progress report helps meet the deadlines and increases the output of the lab. It also helps in knowing what is going on and where one can need help in his/her work. The weekly update turns the actions into accomplishments. Preparing a weekly report is one of the successful habits for many research labs. It will also help in the preparation of experiments planned for the progress of the work. Further, having knowledge and information regarding lab mates' work, experiments having the same material and method (RT-PCR, Gel Electrophoresis, etc.) can be planned and can be run together to save time and chemicals. This will also help in the timely analysis and compilation of the experiments.

12.11 Role of Yoga in Better Understanding and Communication

Yoga helps in better understanding and communication, because it has an immense power to relax the mind, increase body awareness and relieve stress. It focuses on the anatomy of the body psychologically and physiologically [22]. A positive attitude, organized thinking, and logical approach come naturally to a yoga learner. Yoga practiced daily gives one a disciplined approach towards work and life. To inculcate Yoga and meditation into the students' routine by a practical approach will help in better understanding, self-regulation, mindfulness, stress reduction, communication and will improve their academic performance. The Yoga protocols must be considered in orientation programs for new students in order for them to have peace from within and to help them lead a stress-free life even with a busy laboratory schedule. Many studies have reported that Yoga helps in focusing and in improving communications skills, performance, sleep quality, and stress reduction in the students who practice Yoga every day [23]. Some stretching and loosening exercises can be practiced during work. For relaxation, a small meditation break can be done. Practicing Yoga together provides synchronization and team experience. Practicing yoga together teaches teamwork ability to manage stress, patience, and adaptability.

12.12 Future Directions and Clinical Implications

This chapter explains how the communication barriers between students and the PI can be overcome by implementing GLP in research laboratories. Orientations, meetings, and communication strategies have been described in a systematic way in this chapter, which may be used as a template to administer in new laboratories or in already established laboratories to train new students and employees so that the clinical translation can be successful.

12.13 Conclusion

Well-defined communications, well-explained orientations, and regular lab meetings play a pivotal in building the GLP in a research laboratory. These ensure the management, progress, and success of the lab and keep the researchers' morale up.

From time-to-time, supervising officials and guides help in establishing and maintaining a cordial relationship with others at work. All the seminars, workshops, orientation programs, refresher courses, poster presentations help in exchanging novel ideas between the lab mates, and the timely appreciation of the result-oriented researches induces the zeal to work more efficiently.

Orientation and meetings are important tools to make a beginner understand about work and the workplace, in which lab meetings and communications act as catalysts to keep a student oriented about their goals. Therefore, time-to-time orientations, regular lab meetings, and continuous communication collectively serve as paramount factors of GLP. This will make great development in improving the student's learning experience.

References

1. Allen TJ, Fustfeld AR. Research laboratory architecture and the structuring of communications. R&D Manag. 1975;5(2):153–64.
2. World Health Organization. Good laboratory practice training manual: for the trainee: a tool for training and promoting good laboratory practice (GLP) concepts in disease endemic countries. World Health Organization; 2010.
3. Wedlich RC, Pires A, Fazzino L, Fransen JM. Good laboratory practice. Part 3. Implementing good laboratory practice in the analytical lab. J Chem Educ. 2013;90(7):862–5.
4. Egbert MM. Scientists' orientation to an experimental apparatus in their interaction in a chemistry lab. Issues Appl Linguist. 1991;2(2).
5. Dreyfus SE, Dreyfus HL. A five-stage model of the mental activities involved in directed skill acquisition. California Univ Berkeley Operations Research Center; 1980.
6. Castells M. Communication power. Oxford: OUP; 2013.
7. Lippi G, Mattiuzzi C. Critical laboratory values communication: summary recommendations from available guidelines. Ann Transl Med. 2016;4(20).
8. Thompson DR, Chappell MF. Communication and representation as elements in mathematical literacy. Read Writ Q. 2007;23(2):179–96.
9. Kumar S, Lata P. Communication skills. New Delhi: Oxford University Press; 2011.
10. Doumont J-L. Creating effective presentation slides; 2007.
11. Buckley K, Karr S, Nisly SA, Kelley K. Evaluation of a mock interview session on residency interview skills. Curr Pharm Teach Learn. 2018;10(4):511–6.
12. Hinde RA. Non-verbal communication. New York: Cambridge University Press; 1972.
13. Wharton T. Pragmatics and non-verbal communication. New York: Cambridge University Press; 2009.
14. Sless D. Learning and visual communication. London: Halsted; 1981.
15. Miller JG. Hedging the master schedule. In: Disaggregation. Springer; 1979. p. 237–56.
16. Ketch A. Conversation: the comprehension connection. Read Teach. 2005;59(1):8–13.
17. Mudaly V, Singh K. Language: a barrier when teaching and learning business studies. Int J. 2018;74(9/1).
18. David Meier L. The Toyota way fieldbook. Tata McGraw-Hill; 2005.
19. Ravn I, editor. Meetings in organizations: do they contribute to stakeholder value and personal meaning. In: Academy of management annual meeting, Philadelphia, PA; 2007.
20. Müller R, Turner JR. The impact of principal–agent relationship and contract type on communication between project owner and manager. Int J Proj Manag. 2005;23(5):398–403.
21. Kauffeld S, Lehmann-Willenbrock N. Meetings matter: effects of team meetings on team and organizational success. Small Group Res. 2012;43(2):130–58.

22. Salmon P, Lush E, Jablonski M, Sephton SE. Yoga and mindfulness: clinical aspects of an ancient mind/body practice. Cogn Behav Pract. 2009;16(1):59–72.
23. Conboy LA, Noggle JJ, Frey JL, Kudesia RS, Khalsa SBS. Qualitative evaluation of a high school yoga program: feasibility and perceived benefits. Explore. 2013;9(3):171–80.

Role of Data Digitization on Data Integrity

13

Kanupriya Sharma, Vyas M. Shingatgeri, and Surinder Pal

13.1 Introduction

Data integrity is defined as the form of data in which it is accurate, complete, consistent, trustworthy, traceable, permanent, and available throughout its lifecycle. Data integrity provides confidence and assurance that the data is generated in compliance with applicable dynamic standards. Data integrity includes prompt, diligent, and legible data recording, which allows data to be valid and accurate. Inadequate records can develop difficulty in generating project outcomes, cause rejections in research publications, and delay the patent filing process. Adopting quality systems in research will motivate one to follow GLP (Good Lab Practices) principles which are the virtues of good science. As stated by NIH that "Good science requires good record keeping which promotes both accountability and integrity in research" [1]. Data integrity, the most essential and critical component of the quality system, can only be ensured by a mechanism in which the scientific data is captured promptly, diligently, and appropriately documented, stored, witnessed, and archived safely and securely.

K. Sharma
Neuroscience Research Lab, Department of Neurology, Post Graduate Institute of Medical Education and Research, Chandigarh, India

V. M. Shingatgeri (✉)
School of Biosciences, Apeejay Satya University, Gurugram, Haryana, India
e-mail: vyas.ms@asu.apeejay.com

S. Pal
Centre for Systems Biology and Bioinformatics, Panjab University, Chandigarh, India

A. Anand (ed.), *Quality Assurance Implementation in Research Labs*,
https://doi.org/10.1007/978-981-16-3074-3_13

A survey by Nature in 2016 reported that in biology alone, over 70% of the researchers were unable to reproduce studies of other scientists, and about 60% were not able to reproduce their own findings [2]. One of the major drawbacks of lack of research reproducibility is the insufficiency of access to raw data, methodological details, and research material [3]. The reasons attributed to this could be improper documentation, not following the standard operating procedures (SOPs), either due to lack of it or for insecurity induced by competition. However, it should be noted that this can be avoided only if the organization sets in good quality systems rather than depending on individuals. Certainly, the scientific knowledge is of immense importance but if the same is not documented as per the quality systems, then this will lead to the repeatability of the similar experiments that were done and standardized by the previous researchers and would lead to the failure as mentioned above. Hence, the quality of data certainly depends on the systems adopted. Thus, GLP principles, if followed in a research lab or made obligatory, will certainly minimize data integrity issues, and data can be handled efficiently by following various mechanisms to identify and eliminate the age-old practices that have affected this. Therefore, this necessitates a GLP system wherein all the studies/research are performed in an organized fashion with thorough planning, with a diligent and prompt recording, appropriately reporting with the amendments made or deviation with proper documentation, and securely archived or stored.

GLP for non-clinical labs has been developed with guidelines set by the OECD and the FDA in federal regulations [4]. GLP refers to a management system to ensure that experiments and operations provide reliable, consistent, and reproducible results under safe conditions. Implementation of GLP in research labs would be a great initiative as one of the fundamental purposes of GLP is to promote the quality and integrity of data in experiments and research by encompassing who, what, when, how, and where of a research experiment.

With the advancement of information technology, the integration of digitalization into the laboratory is also flourishing. Data digitization can be defined as the processes which are required to manage the data into digital format, whether the digitally generated data, i.e., acquired directly (e.g., email, word doc, excel spreadsheet, e forms, etc.) or has been transformed from hardcopy (e.g., scanned documents). Data digitization can improve the efficiency of processes involved in maintaining data integrity like capturing documents and data at the point of origin, eliminating transcription errors, implementation of electronic workflow processes, creation of audit trials, implementation of security protocols, creation of one source of data for each document, improvement of accessibility of information and also the integration of quality systems from top to bottom. The primary purpose of digitization is to ensure a solution that would bring significant improvements in productivity and quality. Of course, regular monitoring of the processes and systems goes without saying.

This chapter discusses integrating the quality system (GLP) with a special reference to data digitization in academic research through the data management tools that maintain data integrity.

13.2 Data in a GLP Lab

Studies or experiments can be invalidated solely on the laboratory's deficiency to adequately and honestly document experimental studie's conduct. This makes it necessary to operate a laboratory under GLP regulatory requirements to ensure quality by adequately identifying, recording, and retaining the data to ensure integrity. As an old thumb rule says, "if you did not write it down, you could not claim to have measured it," which applies to how, where, and what is required to be written down to claim to have measured it. In other words, "if you have not documented, then you have not done"/OR "If there is no documentation, things have not happened."

Enormous data is being generated in any research laboratory. Hence, it becomes an essential task to manage the same for a meaningful outcome, and this is possible only when the data set is consistent, accurate, and appropriately documented to provide confidence and ensure repeatability and reproducibility. Thus, if the research labs are also operated under GLP, the raw data and the metadata generated will be trustworthy, dependable, and reliable. This is because the documented data covers all the processes, not limited to the record of the chemical receipt or to the usage of the instruments at the time of the experiment. Following GLP principles ensures every step's documentation, right from planning to the performance, that encompasses recording, reporting, monitoring, and archiving. Every step in the process is defined so that the amendments are made on a scientific basis or otherwise, and if the deviations occur, these are recorded with reason and impact, if any, on the outcome. Thus, GLP encourages researchers to organize their work and perform in a way that promotes the good quality, science, and validity of the data generated. Therefore, it requires every researcher to be responsible/accountable for the organization and the work undertaken and the data generated in compliance with GLP so that the data generated is reliable, repeatable, auditable, and recognized globally by the scientific community. Figure 13.1 provides a schematic of what and how data is recorded in a GLP compliant lab.

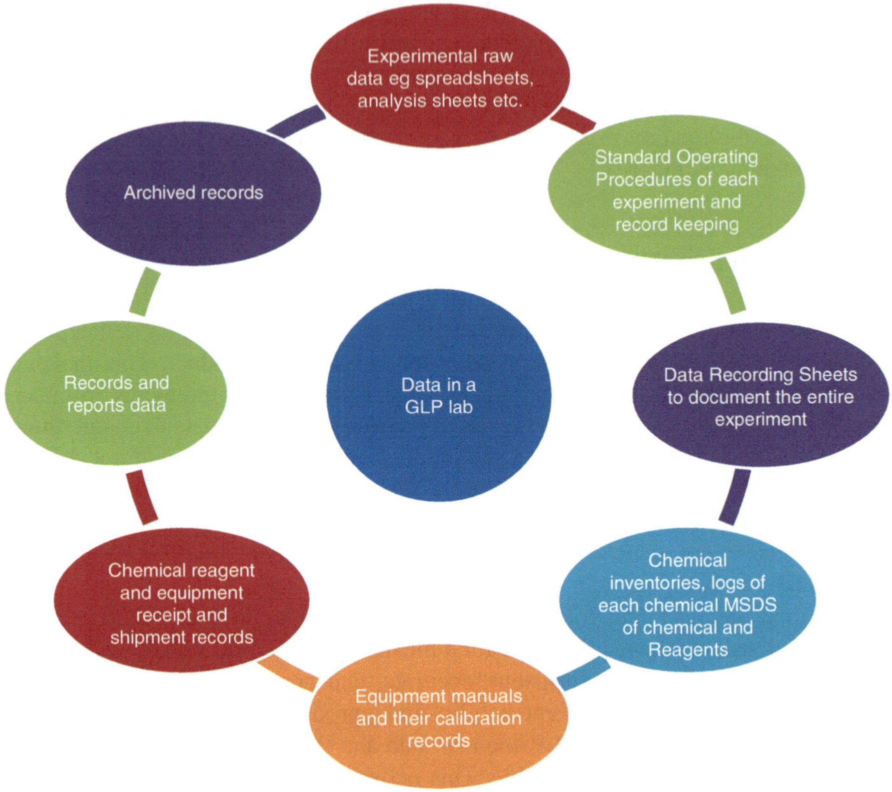
Experimental raw data eg spreadsheets, analysis sheets etc.
Standard Operating Procedures of each experiment and record keeping
Data Recording Sheets to document the entire experiment
Chemical inventories, logs of each chemical MSDS of chemical and Reagents
Equipment manuals and their calibration records
Chemical reagent and equipment receipt and shipment records
Records and reports data
Archived records
Data in a GLP lab

Fig. 13.1 Type of data generated in a GLP compliant lab. Maintenance of data in this format allows easier and convenient workflow in a laboratory. GLP documentation practices also generate enough evidence of the data to ensure its integrity and reliability. GLP, good lab practices

13.3 Life Cycle of Data

Data is the most valuable resource and hence an asset of research. The various sequence of stages from the initial generation to its archival defines the life cycle of data, Fig. 13.2 shows the various stages of the life cycle of data. The cycle starts with the generation of data, followed by data collection, not all the data created is collected defining a filter on the data that we generate, this is a real challenge as huge data is generated and organized, and analyzed to arrive at a logical conclusion which requires efficient data management. In the process of data generation, there is every chance of losing an important aspect of the data, and, therefore, data integrity, being an essential component of the quality system, ensures reliability. The data collected is then processed, including several steps from cleaning, formatting, data compression for efficient storage, data translation for the conversion of paper/

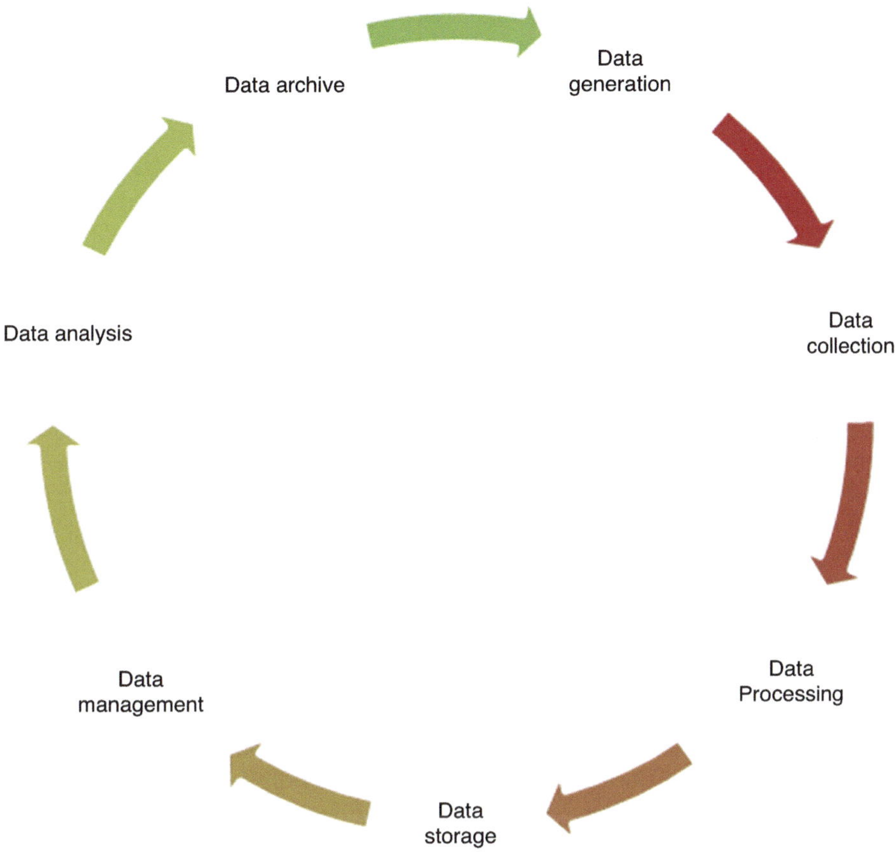
Data archive
Data generation
Data collection
Data Processing
Data storage
Data management
Data analysis

Fig. 13.2 Life cycle of data in an academic research lab

document data into digital form, and data encryption for security. After processing, the same needs to be stored and organized; storage is made as bits of data converted into memory for efficient retrieval. After storage data has to be managed into different data types, depending on its heterogeneity, increase the ability to access and modify data for subsequent analysis, including the statistical techniques or algorithms applied to interpret inferences from the data. A scientist could make a new discovery; a new policy could be developed for the community's future. These inferences could help in the advancement of research and development. After the inferences being drawn from it, it must be archived to ensure its integrity and replicability. Each phase of the data lifecycle is crucial for data integrity. Most research labs do not have a stringent rule for maintaining data, which questions the data generated and published by these labs. Following GLP guidelines in research labs would ensure the reliability of the data generation process, and this would also prevent data falsification and manipulation practices at any stage of the data life cycle.

The entire lifecycle of data highlights the importance of using data responsibly, addressing privacy and ethical concerns. Loss of data and data integrity infringement may occur during the data life cycle due to the following conditions:

- Human error
- Usage of a non-validated computer system to acquire and process data
- Lack of adequate review of original records and data
- GLP-based principles are required to be followed to overcome these shortcomings of data

13.4 Principles of Data Integrity

Good Documentation Practices are essential to ensure data integrity, a fundamental component of GLP compliant research lab [5]. The fundamental principles for maintaining data, either electronic or paper-based, are summarized by the acronym ALCOA and ALCOA+. Table 13.1 summarizes the ALCOA and ALCOA+ acronyms [6]:

ISO (International Organization for Standardization) based recommendations on digitization of data: ISO/TR 13028:2010 [7] in the year 2010 recommended guidelines for digitizing records for establishing standard maintaining records digitally, which were developed to be used by all the organizations to undertake digitization process for record management purposes.

ISO 13008:2012 [8] in the year 2012 ISO specified the planning issues, requirements, and procedure for converting and migration of digital records keeping the authenticity, reliability, integrity, and usability of the documents, which guides to convert records from hardware to software configuration.

Table 13.1 Tabular representation of principles of data integrity ALCOA and ALCOA+ as proposed by FDA

Principle	Meaning
Attributable	The source data is identifiable: who/when created a record and who/when/ why changed a record
Legible	Information is clear and readable
Contemporaneous	Data is recorded at the time of data generation and/or event
Original/True copy	Availability of source information in its original and true form
Accurate	No errors and editing without documented amendments

ALCOA+	Meaning
Complete	Data is recorded, including repeat and reanalysis performed
Available	Availability and accessibility of the data at any time for review or audit and for the lifetime of the data
Consistent	Constant application of harmonized documentation
Enduring	Retrievability of data during its entire lifetime

13.5 Need of Digital Transformation

Researchers' fundamental obligation is to ensure data integrity by maintaining the verifiable accuracy of data, analyses, and conclusions. It has been surveyed that many of the researchers and academicians fail to provide the complete raw data of their findings when asked for [9]. This clearly indicates either the data has not been generated or is not available, and this brings in the credibility of the researchers and highlights the integrity of the data generated in academic research. Thus, it brings a pertinent point of appropriate training of the researchers and understands the importance of the quality systems in academic research to improve credibility and acceptance. It is agreed that every researcher has great in-depth scientific knowledge but fails to understand that GLP brings in good science in whatever efforts and hard work in academic research. Though good documentation practices are considered a burden, it is an essential component of GLP as it brings in greater transparency and helps one introspect and identify the exact reason behind the failure to achieve the objectives despite sincere efforts. Such training can be digitally facilitated by a learning management system that trains and qualifies every researcher on their standard operating procedures and the daily routine. This also ensures when a refresher training needs to be carried out with attending amendments and deviations. GLP system is well established in the commercial labs and a few national test labs, but it is yet to be installed and accepted in research labs and academia. The voluntary establishment of the GLP system in the research lab can bring responsibility and accountability and generate authentic, reliable, consistent, and auditable data, thereby increasing acceptance by the global community. Once the research lab commits to be a GLP system, it will establish the systems and processes that will remain when people move and make things easier to follow to enhance productivity.

Current practices in most laboratories include manual entry or paper data, and hence documentation of such massive data by people can bring in a lot of transcription errors and generate a lot of documents that include all the records right from planning to archiving. Such data is now being converted into electronic data by scanning and storing both physical paper data forms and electronic format. Handling and maintaining documents in a GLP compliant system can be made more comfortable with the implementation of information technology as with the development of cloud computing or similar systems wherein the data can be collected, easily handled, and stored, maintaining its integrity ensuring data security [10]. Digital data also provides easier access to manage and eases its verification, discovery, and evidence generation. However, digitization also combines the challenge of massive data generated, especially in a laboratory where everything is in electronic format and the digital systems directly acquire all the data. This is because the analysis of such data is a huge task and mind-boggling, and needs software that helps make the logical conclusion of the data generated. Addressing these big data analysis issues would also require the regular on-site validation of this software.

13.6 Efficient Digital Data Management Infrastructure

The development of efficient data management infrastructure is an essential aspect of digitization in research. Customized standard procedures need to be developed to digitize different categories of data generated in research, enabling researchers to streamline their research work alongside maintaining the fidelity and quality of research by maintaining data integrity. Below we provide an array of data management infrastructure that constitute the GLP system, and we also discuss the merits of their digitization:

Chemical Log Sheets and Inventory Digitization Inventory maintenance is one of the essential things to run a research lab smoothly. Monitoring the supply of reagents, consumables, lab equipment, and instruments can help check a record of lab requirements, thus increasing productivity and reducing costs.

Figure 13.3 depicts a representation of a log sheet developed for a particular chemical/reagent which is commonly used in research labs.

Merits of Inventory Digitization With all the information about the location, expiry date, lot number, and details about the consumption of reagents and chemicals in an organized system makes it easier to retrieve, restock, and maintain a record of details of consumption of reagents, Fig. 13.4 represents a reference of manual inventory update. Digitized log sheets and inventories on the server, which are accessible to the lab members, allow accessibility to find the product with its location in the defined inventory. Digital update of the inventories allows the user to keep a track of stocking the level and locations of organizing the burden of inventory management.

Temperature Mapping of Ultra-Freezers Preservation of biospecimens in ultra-freezers is considered critical for reliable and reproducible results in genomics, proteomics, and other assays, but their quality can deteriorate with temperature variability within the storage units. Hence ultra-freezers require a daily record of temperature to ensure no temperature variability. However, most of the laboratories use data loggers that provide a good source of information, and all of these are either connected to a building management system that sends alarms to the security officers, the researchers on their cell phone if there in case of emergency.

Merits of Digital Temperature Logs A calibrated digital temperature logger will generate more accurate, useful, and reliable temperature recordings than manual, along with saving time and resources.

e-Lab Notebooks (Electronic Lab Notebooks) Documentation of experiments and their details in the lab is critical and essential for data generation in research. In most of the labs, this is performed on paper notebooks. With digital advancement, e-Lab notebooks have been introduced and currently in use in many GLP laboratories.

Kit log sheets

Lot/Batch No. -	Date of Receiving –
Art no. -	Date of Opening-
Make -	Expiry Date –
Storage -	Quantity -
Total Amount -	

KLS No.	Edition No.01	Effective Date	Review Date	Document Controller (Signature/Stamp)
Copy No.1	Date of Issue	Location (Unit/Division)		

S.No.	Date	User's Name	Use/Project Code	Amt. Used	Bal. Amt.	Sign/ Remarks

Fig. 13.3 Transcript of log sheet developed for a GLP compliant research lab

Merits of e-Lab Notebooks e-Lab notebooks would provide advanced data sharing, flexible lab data organization with easier search through keyword search. Data presentation will also be easier to be understood in the e-Lab notebook format.

Restricted Circulation Photocopying Prohibited

RACK INVENTORY

INVENTORY UPDATE	
Location: Room No.	Month:
Maintained By:	Updated on:

ARRANGED AS PER LIST: A B C →

Chemical No.	Name of the Chemicals	Company	Lot. No./ Batch No.	Quantity	Expiry Date
1.					
2.	Ammonium Persulphate (*Electrophoresis Reagent*)	Sigma	033K1339	15 gm	NA
3.	Ammonium hydroxide solution	Fluka	8314P	1 bottle	NM
4.	Acetonitrile (Expired on 05.04.2009)	Sigma	7352E	1L	05.04.2009
5.	Ammonium molybdate	Sigma	037K01591	100g	NA
6.	Acetic Acid	Sigma	S43484-467	410.3ml	NA
7.	Agarose (Low Melting Point)	Sigma	64H0139	7.70 gm	NA
8.	Activated Charcoal Norit	Fluka	412540/1	250 gm	NA
9.	L-Ascorbic acid (Vitamin C)	Sigma	10H-05545	100 gm	NA
10.	Ammonium Chloride	Sigma	097K07131	470.34 gm	NA
11.	Ammonium Chloride (In 50ml tubes)- To be discarded	SD Fine		2 Tubes	
12.	Ammonia Solution	Merck	HH8H580700	400ml	NM

Chemical Inventory

Fig. 13.4 The manual inventory update followed in a GLP compliant research lab. In a research lab, inventories can be managed by students by performing the role of the store in charge for the smooth functioning of the lab. Regular updates and management of inventory are required to be done with review by QA and Management

Camera Recordings Video recordings provide the origin of data, which otherwise cannot be ensured as it is only known to the user present at the time of experiment and knows about the source of data.

Merits of Camera Recordings Camera surveillance with equipment/instrument accompanying the primary data validates the data origin process, which could be an alternative to manual inspection.

Master Schedule Master schedule is the planning of tasks and experiments into scheduled charts and details. Anticipated planning of the tasks allows smooth workflow and is also a guide for the laboratory in charge or the supervisor who has access to this to evaluate the workload and understand how much can be achieved in a given period and what needs to be done to provide help if deemed essential. This becomes handy for the researchers to promptly complete the task and allows them to document the reasons if things are pending and are not completed.

Merits of Digital Master Schedule Digital master schedule would allow the lab members to access other lab members' master schedules and plan their work in an extremely convenient manner allowing the experiments to be completed smoothly in a planned program. Digital access to other lab member's master schedule allows planning to be more precise as this would avoid overlap of timings for equipment usage. For example, if one lab member has planned his/her experiment on the use of the florescent microscope for a particular date and time, others in the lab can plan their work as per this schedule so that there is no overlap of timings and interruption at that time.

Master Coding Master codes are like a barcode of a document, specimen, or sample. They are developed to identify the location of the sample/ document, sample disease, personnel responsible for that document/ sample. They are actually considered a sample characterization document and provide all the relevant and useful data for the researchers. Figure 13.5 depicts a sample master coding as a reference for a research lab.

Merits of Digital Master Coding A standard digital interface of the master coding format would allow the lab members to identify a coded sample or document without going through the pages of documents to scroll down its identity. It also helps in using the right model for an appropriate experiment and its identification.

Chemical/Reagent/Equipment Receipt and Shipment Record A record of receipt and shipment must be maintained to verify the goods' receipt and ascertain its shelf life. They can be placed at their desired locations in order Logbook and log sheets are developed as is applicable for resources utilized in the laboratory, including the equipment, machinery, pipettes, etc.

MASTER CODING

Species

1. HUMAN
2. MICE
   STRAIN
3. RAT
   STRAIN
4. MONKEY

Disease/Sample Type (Human)

01. PARKINSON'S DISEASE
02. ARMD
03. ALS
04. STROKE
05. ALZHEIMER DISEASE
06. ATAXIA'S
07. MUSCULAR DYSTROPHY
08. TUBERCULOSIS MENINGITIS
09. NEUROCYSTICERCOSIS
10. RETINAL DEGENERATION
11. SPINO MUSCULAR DYSTROPHY
12. FAMILIAL HEMIPLEGIC MIGRAINE
13. LEUKODYSTROPHY
14. DOPA RESPONSIVE DYSTONIA
15. FRONTOTEMPORAL DEMENTIA
16. PICK'S DISEASE
17. CORTICO-BASAL DEGENERATION
18. PROGRESSIVE SUPRANUCLEAR PALSY
19. NEUROFIBROMATOSIS TYPE 1 & 2
20. MENTAL RETARDATION 1
21. WILSON DISEASE
22. X-LINKED MENTAL RETARDATION AND MICPCH
23. FRAGILE X SYNDROME AND MANTEL RETARDATION
24. CHARCOT-MARIE-TOOTH DISEASE
25. DYSLEXIA
26. EPILEPSY
27. ANEUPLOIDY
28. PRENATAL MICRO DELETION SYNDROME
29. ANTERIOR CRUCIATE LIGAMENT (ACL)
30. HUNTINGTON DISEASE
31. YOGA
32. SPINAL CORD INJURY
33. PRE DAIBETIC
34. ORAL CANCER

Disease MODEL (ANIMAL)

GLOBAL	01
MCAO	02
NMDA	03
LASER	05
6-OHDA	06
MEMORY-AB	07
PPA	08
OPTIC NERVE CRUSH	09

Categories in animal/human sample
Human sample:
A- TEST (A_1=PRE; A_2=POST),
B -NORMAL CONTROL,
C- NEUROLOGICAL CONTROL;
Animal sample:

A- CONTROL
B- DISEASE
C- DISEASE+ VEHICLE
D- DISEASE+ TREATMENT
E- SHAM CONTROL
F- PER SE

Form of Disease

FOR EXAMPLE
JUVENILE: α
YOUNG:β
ADULT ONSET: φ
LATE ONSET:$
SPORADIC: *
FAMILIAL: #

Patient/ Sample Number
001-999
Follow Up Sample Number
F001-F999

TYPE OF SAMPLE
01: PLASMA
02: SERUM
03: LYMPHOCYTES
04: DNA
05: RNA
06: PCR PRODUCTS
07: cDNA
08: CSF SAMPLE
09: BIOPSY SAMPLES
10: AUTOPSY SAMPLES
11: VITEROUS
12. HOMOGENATE
13. CELL LINE

ALIQUOTS
A,B,C,D

SCHOLARS
01: ABC
02: DEF
03: GHI

Fig. 13.5 A sample of master coding of various kinds of samples being used in a research lab

Merits of Digital Receipt and Shipment Record A digital record of lab consumables provides access and updates to each of the lab members about every new chemical's receipt and location. Digital record-keeping of every minor use of chemicals/reagents is also maintained digitally on a more manageable platform. This is mainly for resource-starved labs.

13.7 Paper to Bits: Conversion of Paper Documents into Digital

Digitization is a digital transformation process where data can be recorded into discrete binary units of bits and can be accessed through computers without much hindrance. The handling and storage of paper and documents manually are difficult and is more prone to damage! Translation of paper documents into digital format needs to follow some standards and steps to ensure the integrity of documents during their digital transformation.

Steps of digitization processes for paper documents:

- Selection and preparation of documents for digitization: Documents are first selected and separated with documents for their specified folders. Records can be images, videos, papers, camera recordings, etc.
- Conversion of information in digital format: After the selection, the document has to be converted into the digital format using a scanner using any computer or mobile scanner to ensure the visibility and readability of the information on the documents.
- Editing, transition, and storage of digitized documents: The documents to be stored have to be saved with the names with which these can be easily identified. Depending upon the format in which the document has to be stored, it should be converted and saved in that format, e.g., pdf, jpeg, tiff, zip files. Folders and files have to be specified for each document with a proper name and storage path.
- Archiving and coding the documents: Archiving is done to ensure the record-keeping for a more extended period. Digital archiving is an essential task in preserving data and thus requires appropriate technical measures to be followed. The archive data should be coded and archived to ensure data privacy.
- QA (Quality Assurance) and validation: Meticulous QA and verification are required to ensure the data's standard.
- Organization of digital data into files and folders: Separate files and folders with the distinction of names and types of data being stored in each file should be maintained. The data has to be organized systematically.
- Access and maintenance: Access to the data can be limited or restricted to the concerned person or depending upon the data type. To ensure data privacy, the folders can be password protected with access provided to authorized individuals only.

As per CGMP guidelines for record-keeping of electronic records, it has to be decided in advance which documents have to be kept in digital or paper format. Based on the decision, it has to be documented either in the form of a Standard Operating Procedure (SOP) or a specified document [11].

13.8 Steps of Digital Transformation

Digital transformation refers to digital documentation and data archive. Both digital and paper form of data has to undergo specific steps for its change into the digital library or storage. These steps have to be followed to keep the data integrity intact.

For a lab to transmute into the digital platform, the data is stored at different places and sites have to be collected at the common repository keeping the data integrity in place. A stepwise procedure has to be developed as discussed below to transform into a digital lab:

Below we discuss the various steps involved in the digital data transformation; Fig. 13.6 represents a flowchart representation of steps involved in the digitization of data:

- Planning: The plan needs to cover the following details: level of scanning required, discrete data that has to be extracted, storage of physical data after digitization, and also the management of scanning of documents.

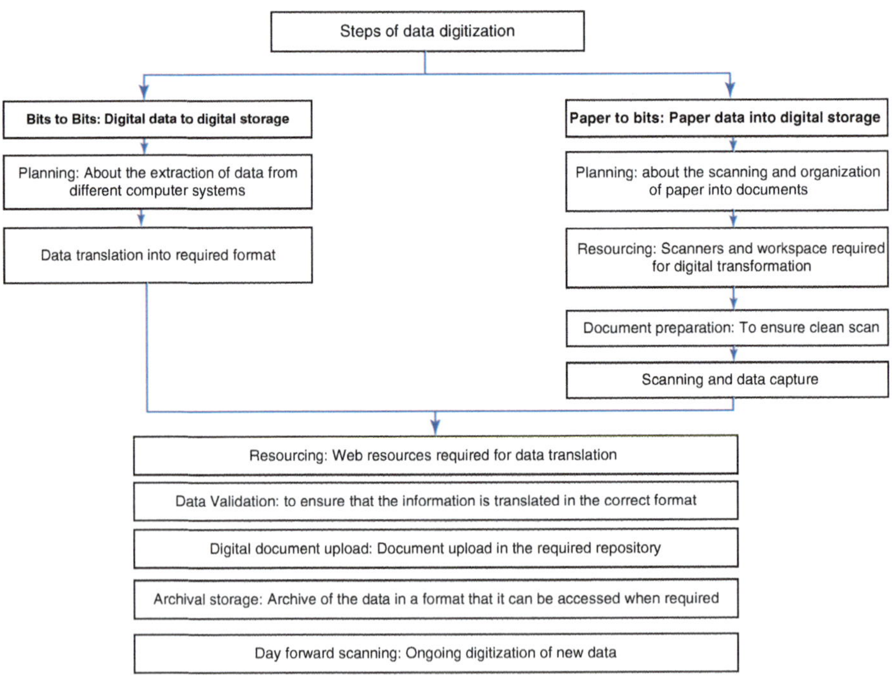

Fig. 13.6 Flowchart representation of data digitization, digitization of both digital data and paper or document-based data

- Resourcing: Workspace, scanners, and other web resources are required.
- Document preparation: Preparation of documents to ensure clean scans of the documents.
- Scanning and data capture: Capture images and discrete data.
- Data validation: Validation of data after conversion would ensure the correct and accurate data transformation procedure.
- Digital document upload: Loading of documents into the required repository of choice.
- Archival storage: Return of digital documents to active storage or deposition when required.
- Day forward scanning: Ongoing digitization of new documents to keep compliance with digital record-keeping.
- Data must be generated to reconstruct proper validation and use of the computerized system. Data must have a risk assessment, supplier assessment, service level agreements, requirement specifications, test records, personnel and user training, change, and configuration records. Documentation and records of validation and use of the specific computerized system should be available as long as the data generated with the system have to be archived as per applicable regulations. As per OECD guidelines for the application of GLP systems to a computerized system, for the documentation of the usage of automated systems for record-keeping and document records, SOP's should be developed which should cover the following points [12]:
  - Procedure for operation of computerized system and responsibilities of personnel involved.
  - Procedure for security measures to detect and prevent unauthorized access.
  - Procedure for periodic testing for the correct functioning of the complete system.
  - Procedure for preventive maintenance and fault repair.
  - Back up procedures.
  - Procedures for archival and retrieval of all documents, software, and computer data.
  - Monitoring and auditing of computerized system.

13.9 Digitization Systems/Equipment's/Components

As digital equivalents replace traditional data saving methods, various systems and equipment have been developed for this purpose; Fig. 13.7 represents server-based GLP system for data handling and data maintenance. The choice of storage solution needs to account for the following points:

Redundancy Data backup must be ensured so that it allows access to the data in any case of system breakdown.

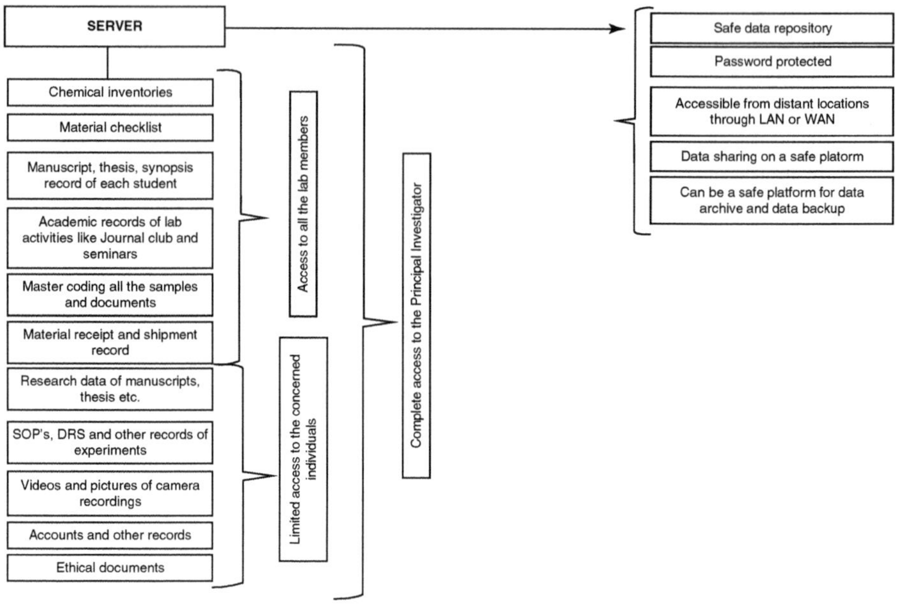

Fig. 13.7 Representation of a server system in a GLP compliant research lab for data handling and data maintenance

Persistence and Preservation Data needs to be tested periodically and fixed if a problem arises as data might get corrupted on the local storage devices, e.g., hard disks become demagnetized rendering it for data disruption.

Transformation With regular advancement in the data storage systems, it should be allowed to migrate data to the latest technological requirements, ensuring that data is not semantically modified or lost while being transformed.

Various digital systems can be used in digitization to establish data integrity by assuring data storage, safety, and security:

- **Barcode:** Barcode recognition can help in the conversion of batches of paper documents into electronic format. Barcodes are inserted at the beginning of each group of files which acts as a guide for recognizing each group of documents. Document management system reads the information in the barcode and manages the batch by establishing an automated system, indexing it, identifying the document type, converting the format, assigning a specific path within the repository, etc.
- **Server:** Server is a computer hardware or software that provides functionality to different computers or clients. These provide functionalities such as sharing data or resources among multiple clients or to perform the computation for a client.
- **Web Repository:** Web repositories are available to access the documents on remote web servers. The documents are made available through content management resources which allows the documents to be indexed and searched. Once

the indexing of the documents is done, it can be assessed through search or browsing taxonomies.

- **Lab Management Software (LMS)** [13]**:** LMS is designed to support the management of data related to biology labs, clinical trials, etc. LMS supports laboratory operations, including management of workflow, data tracking support, data exchange interface, and many more. Additional features provided by LMS include sample management, data exchange, audit management, barcode handling, compliance (following regulatory standards), document management, a record of instrument calibration, inventory management, quality assurance, and traceability of samples and audit trails.
- **Inventory control management system** [14] provides the stock details in a web-based repository management system that manages the stock usage or balance of chemicals and reagents based on barcodes and QR codes that are linked to the database. By scanning the QR code or barcode, automatic update with the name of the student or person who used the chemical is updated on the online inventory. This eases the process of audit for auditors to generate track of the used and stock chemicals and reagents.

Digital Risks

Adoption of digital technologies can have new and unexpected consequences. Below discussed are some of the risks associated with the digital transformation [15]:

- Risk of cybersecurity: Cyberattacks are done with the objective to access information. Cyberattacks make the data prone to loss and misuse.
- Skill shortage: Shortage of skills among the lab members to use the digital interface.
- Compliance risk: Standards of GLP which are followed manually might not be followed with the digital transformation.
- Resilience risk: Risk of negative events occurring at the time of switching to digital technology can lead to data loss.

Mitigation of Digital Risks

- Limited access to the digital repository and blocking of the domains and IP addresses using firewalls, proxy, or perimeter controls.
- Training to the lab individuals about the usage of the digital interface should be provided before joining into the digital system.
- QA personnel should be well informed about the usage and importance of digital systems. QA should ensure compliance with the GLP standards by making regular audit trails.

In case of negative events or breakdown of the system, data backup acts as the raw data resource.

13.10 Data Security

In the digital age, digital security is essential for the maintenance of data security as digital data is prone to malware. Data encryption, the firewall is data classification systems that provide data security provision.

- **Data Encryption:** With encryption, data can be translated into a code called ciphertext. Only authorized users with private decryption keys are allowed to decrypt the encrypted data.
- **Use of Original Software:** The use of pirated software is likely to have serious viruses, damaging the computer system, and the data can be lost. The use of pirated software can also be a risk for data security. Illegal usage of pirated software is also against copyright infringement law. Hence, to ensure data security use of original software is mandatory.
- **Firewall Security:** The firewall establishes a predetermined security system that monitors and controls the incoming and outgoing network traffic. It creates a barrier between the internal network from external internet sources. Firewall analyze incoming network based on pre-established rules and filter traffic coming from unsecured or suspicious sources. Network-based firewalls can be positioned between LAN (Local Area Network) or WAN (Wide Area Network). Through LAN, data can be accessed by the local IP addresses, and through WAN, it allows distant network zones to access through the server. Through a firewall, accessibility to the server can be restricted to identified IP addresses.
- **Cloud Data Storage:** Cloud data storage is a user-friendly, low expenditure method for data storage. This does not occupy any hardware space. Cloud data storage provides outsourcing of data storage, which minimizes data loss as the data storage administrator offers security and storage responsibility. At the time of processing the data, a private key is used to retrieve the stored data. Files and folders can be password protected in a cloud-based data storage system. Data auditing can be done through the multi-level tree algorithm. For an internal GLP protocol, a high-security cloud-based system can be installed which provides data security, storage, and retrieval at the time of need.

13.11 Expenses in Digitization Process

The initial digital transformation would incur cost investments to leverage a combination of data, computing, and connecting technologies. With all the advantages of digital transformation and cost investments, its benefits cannot be ignored. Understanding the amount of the data generated, handling the same, and carrying out the operating processes in a laboratory would either require hiring the resources or do many things and may end up with the data that cannot be analyzed consistently. Therefore, adapting to digitization is the only answer to acquire and capture the data enabling the research laboratory to generate accountable and consistent data.

Connecting a lab to a digital data management system is more dependable in the long term, but initial investments are required. However, the expenses curve falls after the initial installation, and the data integrity curve rises.

Below listed include a few expenses but not limited to be considered in the digitization procedure:

- Installation of system which can be a common digitization platform with secure access to the allowed lab members.
- Installation of high-resolution cameras for video recording at the site of data generation.
- Scanners and printers linked with LAN to allow limited and secure access.
- Barcode inventory management software installation.
- Biometric/ fingerprint scan to digitize the use of an instrument while performing any experiment.

While the improvised process would incur cost but it is worthwhile as it would add value to the systems and process, and in long run, it not only provides credibility but also improves efficiency and lowers the overall cost. Moreover, the cost can be spread for a year or 2, depending on the priority, and with proper care and planning, the entire cost can be recovered with what the research lab will achieve with the digitized quality system. Further, the cost incurred will allow the digitized system as a tool for the management to monitor the resources more effectively and take an appropriate action either to amend certain activities that are not yielding results and are still incurring cost or divert the resources as deemed essential. Digital transformation would certainly involve investments, but if done at the right time, by taking a calculated risk of the resources versus the quality, it would help be beneficial. While installation of the equipment's for direct data capture is useful, a few dedicated to transforming the existing data to the digital format can be planned in a prudent manner. Digital transformation can be initiated in processes by following digitization activities like document capture through scanning, document capture through e forms, the capture of metadata, identifying printed characters using photoelectric devices and computer software to avoid data entry (personal errors as a result of data entry) to systems, creating workflow functions to automate control process by providing authorization and creating the audit trails, using learning management systems to recognize the versions and control of the versions, emailing attachments using electronic signatures/encrypting and eliminating the security issues can be considered to merge in a best possible way to avoid repetitions.

These things help to reduce unnecessary repetitions, which are done manually. The goal of transforming to digital data capture and reporting method is to avoid the transcription errors, and the huge errors committed while making manual entry and reduce the amendments and deviations as well as objection from auditors and regulators. Further, this ensures seamless access of data to research scientists working in the laboratory who otherwise tend to rely on their memory. Digitization brings challenges in terms of cost, training, huge data analysis, it can be effectively implemented by proper planning and implementation in order to bring value addition and efficiency in the organization and effectively reducing the overall costs in the long run.

13.12 Data Integrity Through Data Auditing

Data integrity is the completeness, consistency, and accuracy of data assuring that the data is attributable, legible, contemporaneously recorded, original, or a true copy and accurate. Inspections and audits are required to be carried out to identify the facts rather than faults, and hence every scientist should encourage audits for self-improvement. Scientists should bear in mind that it is not a fault-finding mission but rather a corrective and preventive measure that would improve the self and, consequently, the adopted systems and processes. Thus, it becomes helpful to the researcher to monitor/audit the laboratory in charge to own the laboratory's responsibility. While internal and external audits might help in the initial stages, it would be essential to develop a robust system that would allow the internal auditor to do a better and honest job as it is an effort to improvise the laboratory systems and not individual credibility. Data auditing procedures include many things but are not limited to the following, like examining laboratory notebooks and worksheets upon which research publications are based [16]. The auditing of digital data is altogether a different procedure and would require effective training with expertise for different software. While the digital systems can help the researchers understand their own mistakes as the systems have the audit trails, this helps them either investigate the impact on the results generated and take a call whether the experiments required to be repeated with appropriate documentation and authorization. Over the last decade, the advancement in the information technology Computer Assisted Auditing Techniques (CAAT) has been developed to reduce the manual auditing procedures. CAAT helps auditors analyze data to explore and study distinct data sets in auditing processes [17].

13.13 Digital Data Archive and Data Backup

Data backup and archive system should be installed for retention, reconstruction, and disaster recovery. SOPs for data archiving have been generated at various platforms. Data archiving requires specific procedures to be followed concerning the content of the data. The data should be stored, maintaining confidentiality, and it should be stored such that it is traceable. Data archiving comprises of management of electronic records by providing security, authenticity, and integrity for long-term preservation and access. Data archiving feature is offered by various data management systems, which involves storing files in standard file format (.PDF, TIFF, JPEG, ASCII text). This can be easily migrated to a new platform when required without any loss of data and any further costs incurrence to the archive.

Roles and responsibilities of various personnel involved in the process of archiving have been discussed in OECD guidelines for establishment and control of archives in compliance with principles of GLP [12, 18]:

- Study director: The study director has to ensure that all records and data related to the study are transferred to the archive immediately after completion of a study.
- Principal Investigator: Principal Investigator ensures that the records for which he/she is responsible are sent to the study director latest upon completion of the study.
- Archivist: The archivist is responsible for the management, operations, and procedures for archiving following established SOP's and GLP principles.

Archivist ensures the control over access to archive by:

- Orderly storage and retrieval of records.
- Documentation of movement of records in and out of the archive.
- Quality Assurance (QA) personnel: QA person ensures the compliance of GLP principles with all the aspects of archiving.

For the archiving procedures, the following SOPs should be developed:

- Access to archive
- Indexing procedures, including electronic records
- Coding procedure for the archive of the data
- Retention period
- Disposal of archived records and material
- Disaster recovery
- Periodic refreshing of electronic records

Some additional features have to be ensured for the archive of electronic records, which includes the following:

- *Retention period*: With the rapid development of computer technology, the devices used for data storage today may not be available in the future (e.g., diminished usage of floppy disks with time). Hence, the electronic records must be stored in a format that is readable for the duration of the applicable record retention period.
- *Defined Archive Area on a Computerized System:* The computer system or the archive data storage system must have a discrete archive area, with limited access to archivist. The system must be locked so that the data cannot be altered or deleted without detection.
- *Maintenance and Preservation of Electronic Data:* Electronic records are at risk without a preservation process. Procedures should be there to ensure the retention of complete and retrievable information throughout the retention period of the data.

- *Data migration:* Data migration is defined as the transfer of data from one system to another system. If the data migration is necessary, the procedure of migration should be fully documented, ensuring complete and accurate migration of data before it is lost or disposed.

In order to ensure the retention of electronic data, duplication of electronic records can be considered as a part of the archive preservation plan.

Data backup is the copy of the original data which can be used to reproduce the raw data and data sets and for that record of all the experiments performed on the data and all the changes done and is required to be submitted for that the data must be exact, complete, and secure from alteration, inadvertent erasure or loss [19]. The backup file should contain the data in the original format or in a format that is compatible with the original format. Data backup provides a backup to the data in case of loss of original data [20].

Data archive and data backup provide support for the replication of scientific experiments using the same methodology, equipment, and protocols based on which scientific claims are evaluated. It is evident that when replication or reproduction of a study has failed, questions arise on how data has arisen. In that case, the traceability and associated documentation provided the required support and digitized archiving of the study documents, which can be easily accessed even after years of the actual study or experiments.

Implementation of a digital GLP-based system in a research lab would develop a systematic data security system with a systematic procedure of data generation, data archive, and data backup; this system would assist authentic data generation with a smooth workflow.

13.14 Challenges in Data Collection, Digitization, and Maintaining Data Integrity

Data digitization is a reliable method for data integrity and credibility for a long term but implementing this procedure has its own challenges.

- Cameras to witness the data generation at the site of experiments should be high focused and high resolution to ensure enough coverage to witness the experiment being performed. This incurs high-cost investments.
- Its quite likely that data may be lost while the same is being transferred from one equipment to another.
- Digitization of data is prone to transcription errors if manually entered from paper to digital system, hence, there is a need for verification at the time of data transfer.
- Regular update and validation of the software being used for digitization have to be ensured in order to avoid data loss and to ensure compliance to GLP.
- Software and systems are required at the time of acquiring data, storing, and archiving of data. Initial training is required for training in respect of the opera-

tion of the software. Hence digitization procedure is not as much cost-effective to switch over immediately.

- Data legibility which can be defined as the ease to read the data, it has to be ensured while data digitization to maintain its readability and the process of digitization has to be validated, ensuring data's legibility.
- Security procedures should be documented to protect the data from corruption and unauthorized modification or loss. Physical and logical methods like the use of keys, pass cards, personal codes with passwords, biometrics, or restricted access to the computer to ensure the security of the data [12].

With all the challenges, a GLP-based system allows data integrity with the assurance of authenticity and reliability of data generation preventing research frauds and resulting in true research being published.

13.15 Implementation of Data Digitization in a GLP Research Lab to Ensure Data Integrity

Digitization is being employed in the IT sector and companies for the storage of their data. Data digitization offers many benefits like it saves time and money in the long run, provides easier access, easy search, and most importantly increases the security of the data.

In science, experimental observations must be shown to be reproducible in order to be creditable. For generating creditability, the integrity of data should be assured. Digitization offers an easier platform for researchers to improvise new techniques to ensure data integrity, but it also offers easier data manipulating and data falsification techniques.

In order for research and experiments to be credible a GLP-based lab generates enough documents and records to create evidence of the data's integrity. Maintenance of data integrity with GLP guidelines ensures documentation of the entire life cycle of the data. To understand the importance of data integrity, GLP training could help provide the lab members about the need of GLP and implementation of GLP in the research lab, documentation of this training is also essential as per GLP rules.

After the training, for installation of GLP-based computerized systems in a pre-planned manner should be carried out. Documentation is an essential purpose of GLP as it involves documentation of management policies, validation, planning, risk assessment, traceability, archivability, security, and record management. As per GLP guidelines, the documentation of the entire life cycle of all the phases should be done, and this may include purchase, specification, design, development and validation, implementation, operation, etc. The computerized system used for GLP should be developed, validated, and operationalised in accordance with appropriate quality management system to ensure that the system is functioning and being used correctly [12].

With the implementation of GLP practices in research lab, not only the records and documentation of data are regulated but this also develops a work system which makes the workflow easier and systematic. Digitization of GLP-based documents generates data integrity of the research data with easier maintenance of the data providing easier sources of data integrity. Data digitization in a GLP-based laboratory would make the documentation and record-keeping of the entire experiments intact and accurate, keeping steer clarity from data misrepresentation.

13.16 Building the Lab of the Future

A future research lab with the implementation of e data generation is the reach of digital data integrity. A lab that holds the usage and record of instrument use with barcode or biometric face readers, direct transfer of data generated into servers, automated equipment, e-notebooks, voice powered lab assistant for data digitization and many more such features of digital advancement may one day help scientists set up hypothesis and design experimental protocols by comparing and contrasting studies available on databases. Advancement in technologies and digitization can offer researchers data accuracy and data integrity which has never existed before.

13.17 Future Directions and Clinical Implications

Integration of GLP compliant digitization system in research can radically transform the practice of scientific research with an increasing ability to automate scientific discovery processes and can also help regulate and manage the workflow in a systematic and correct manner. Adoption of GLP-based digitization system in research labs can make management productive preventing academic fraud, and this would have direct implications on the clinical research by improving clinical data collection, translation, and record-keeping.

13.18 Conclusion

Adopting GLP principles and adhering to them by research laboratories is the only alternative to bring in quality and data acceptability while avoiding the issues that have been associated with fraudulent practices or data falsification, which is evident once the data is sent for publication to the Journals of repute where in some aspect of auditing or restructuring remotely is being done. GLP is mandatory for the toxicological studies that are required to be submitted for the regulatory approvals as they form the basis for clinical studies and marketing authorization, and hence ensuring safety becomes a key criterion. If the research labs adopt the GLP principles, it must be ensured that all the activities are planned and performed with adherence to a set of formal national and international agreed guidelines established by the said regulatory authorities. In such case, the data generated from a GLP-based research lab will certainly be accountable, auditable and will provide better traceability and reproducibility and thus global acceptability. If the research laboratories adopt the digitization process, it will not only improve the quality and acceptability across the globe but will also help the lab to manage the data efficiently and cost-effectively. Adopting GLP in the research laboratories are yet to be initiated by organizations, the thought process must be initiated in order to gear up for the adoption of GLP principles. Research laboratories can voluntarily adopt to implement GLP modules on a digital interface in their labs which would ensure data integrity, promote high-quality safety and consistency in the processes and thereby increase efficiency.

References

1. NIH. Guidelines for scientific record keeping in the intramural research program at the NIH; 2008. https://oir.nih.gov/sites/default/files/uploads/sourcebook/documents/ethical_conduct/guidelines-scientific_recordkeeping.pdf
2. Baker M. 1,500 scientists lift the lid on reproducibility. Nature. 2016;533(7604):452–4.
3. Dirnagl U. Rethinking research reproducibility. EMBO J. 2019;38(2):e101117.
4. Baldeshwiler AM. History of FDA good laboratory practices. Qual Assur J. 2003;7(3):157–61.
5. Scheme PIC/S. Good practices for data management and integrity in regulated GMP/GDP environments; 2018.
6. McDowall R. Data integrity and data governance: practical implementation in regulated laboratories. Royal Society of Chemistry; 2018.
7. ISO. Information and documentation—implementation guidelines for digitization of records. ISO/TR 13028:2010; 2010.
8. ISO. Information and documentation—digital records conversion and migration process. ISO 13008:2012; 2012.
9. Corbyn Z. Researchers failing to make raw data public. Nature. 2011. https://www.nature.com/news/2011/110914/full/news.2011.536.html.
10. Working Group on Information Technology. Good laboratory practice (GLP); guidelines for the archiving of electronic raw data in a GLP environment. Qual Assur J. 2003;7(4):262–9.
11. FDA. Guidance for industry part 11, electronic records; electronic signatures—scope and application [Internet]; August 2003. https://www.fda.gov/media/75414/download
12. OECD. OECD draft advisory document 16 the application of GLP principles to computerised systems; 2014.
13. Skobelev D, Zaytseva T, Kozlov A, Perepelitsa V, Makarova A. Laboratory information management systems in the work of the analytic laboratory. Meas Tech. 2011;53(10):1182–9.
14. Kagami A, Homma K, Akashi K, Aizawa T, Mori H. Inventory control method and system. Google Patents; 1992.
15. Oliveira Dd. Plutora [Internet]. 2020. https://www.plutora.com/blog/author/danieldeoliveira. Accessed 8 Dec 2020.
16. Glick JL, Shamoo AE. Auditing biochemical research data: a case study. Account Res. 1991;1(4):223–43.
17. Pedrosa I, Costa CJ. Computer assisted audit tools and techniques in real world: CAAT's applications and approaches in context. Int J Comput Inf Syst Ind Manag Appl. 2012;4:161–8.
18. OECD. Establishment and control of archives that operate in compliance with the principles of GLP [Internet]. 2007. http://www.oecd.org/officialdocuments/publicdisplaydocumentpdf/?doclanguage=en&cote=env/jm/mono(2007)10
19. Williams M, Bagwell J, Zozus MN. Data management plans: the missing perspective. J Biomed Inform. 2017;71:130–42.
20. Stiles T. The revised OECD principles of good laboratory practice. A reflection upon the impact the proposed changes will have upon pre-clinical safety testing. Part 2. Qual Assur J. 1997;2(2):49–53.

GPSR Compliance

The European Union's (EU) General Product Safety Regulation (GPSR) is a set of rules that requires consumer products to be safe and our obligations to ensure this.

If you have any concerns about our products, you can contact us on ProductSafety@springernature.com

In case Publisher is established outside the EU, the EU authorized representative is:

Springer Nature Customer Service Center GmbH
Europaplatz 3
69115 Heidelberg, Germany

Batch number: 10583317

Printed by Printforce, the Netherlands